MOUTHBODY HEALTHCARE

The Hidden Link Between Your Dentistry and Chronic Illnesses

Camilla Griggers, PhD

First printing, 2025.

Cover photograph Allef Vinicius on Unsplash.

ISBN-13: 978-1-962984-94-2

Waterside Productions

2055 Oxford Ave
Cardiff, CA 92007

www.waterside.com

Waterside Productions

For my mother and father, Ellen and Victor.

And for Georgena Grace.

Since our orthodox theories [of modern dentistry, medicine and food production] have not saved us, we may have to bring them into harmony with Nature's laws. Nature must be obeyed, not orthodoxy.

—Weston A. Price, DDS, from *Nutrition and Physical Degeneration*

Table Of Contents

Put Your Body Where Your Mouth Is

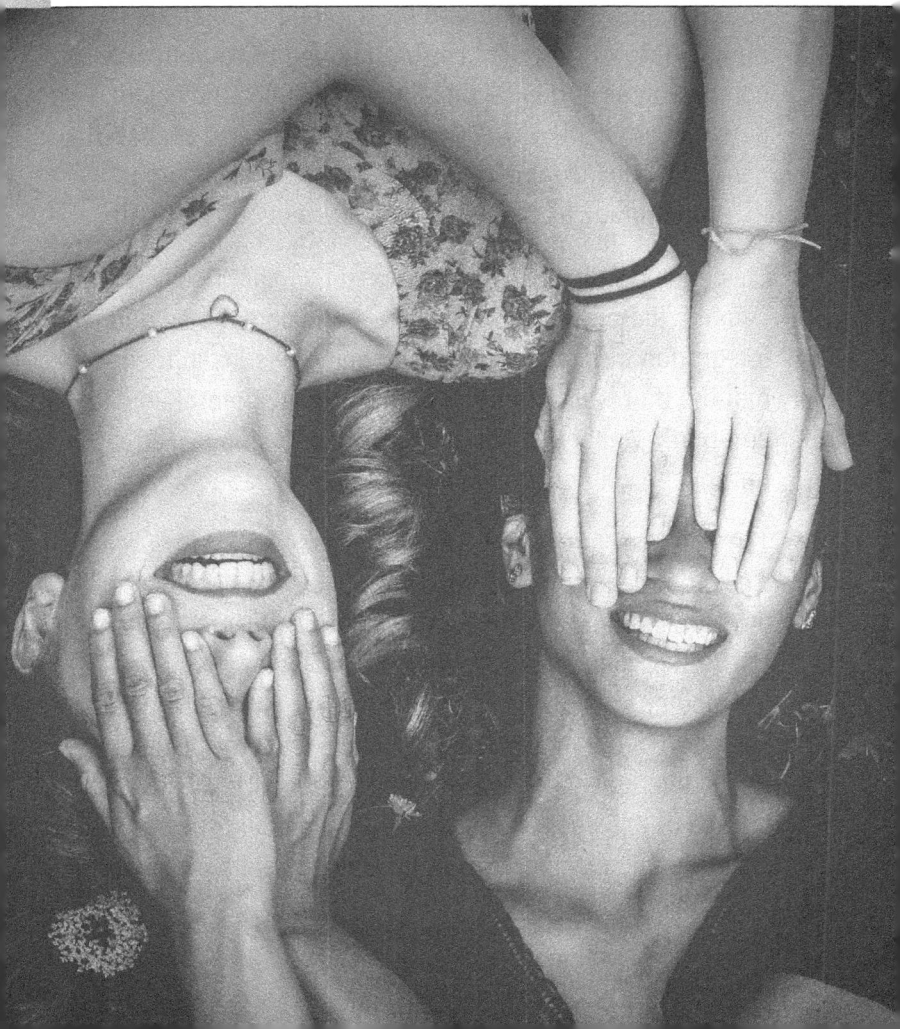

This book was written with the intention to succinctly explain everything you need to know to take care of your mouthbody health now and for the rest of your life. I use the term *mouthbody* to remind you that your mouth is connected to the rest of you!

I know that seems obvious, but accepting the reality of *the mouthbody connection* radically changes the conventional allopathic dentistry that Americans have known in the past, in which invasive treatments could be applied in your mouth with little regard for the long-term effects on your future systemic health. Honoring the mouthbody connection as a foundational principle of holistic health puts modern dentistry in its proper place as one aspect of general medicine. And it helps you put your oral care in its proper place as one aspect of your holistic self-care.

This book began as an informational PDF that I gave to my somatic therapy clients who were doing somatic-emotional integration work and were facing dental issues in their mouths that were affecting their physical, mental and emotional wellbeing. I'm happy the book is now available for anyone who needs the information, because we all do!

The following chapters will help you understand what causes 6 common dental problems that can affect your systemic health, the risks associated with conventional treatments for them, followed by safer prevention-oriented solutions that leverage the mouthbody connection. In the final chapters, I help you jumpstart better mouthbody healthcare and provide resources to find the right dentist for you and your family. My goal by the end of this book is that you have something you can really smile about on Instagram—better lifelong health outcomes!

Mystory

I came to understand the need for a holistic approach to dentistry the hard way—through trial and error and chasing symptoms that resulted in dental trauma that could have been avoided. My mouthbody story began when I was a teenager. My mother took me and my brother to the neighborhood dentist for a cleaning. In spite of the fact that my mother cooked healthy meals for breakfast and dinner and we rarely ate sweets, the regular trips to the dentist for cleanings soon included drilling and filling with mercury amalgam dental fillings. Over time a small filing attracted recurrent decay around the edges and became a larger filling and later larger still.

Twenty years later, I was a young professor at Carnegie Mellon University teaching gender studies, media studies and cultural studies, when I cracked one of those old mercury amalgam fillings on a popcorn kernel. Copying how my busy working mother had chosen our dentist when I was a child, I made an appointment with the dentist closest to my home without a second thought.

On the fateful day of my appointment, the conventionally trained dentist drilled a cracked mercury amalgam filling without protective equipment, spewing mercury vapor and particulate into my mouth, face and lungs. And just like that, off I went down the mercury toxicity rabbit hole. What a trip! At that time, I lacked a basic understanding of what had happened to me and how to help myself recover my health. To top it off, that dentist put a crown on the tooth that was too high (a common occurrence if a dentist isn't trained in structural dentistry), and as a result my jaw was out of alignment for years after, causing headaches and shooting chronic pain down my neck into my shoulder blades.

Some of you may recognize the situation I found myself in. Dental trauma like what I experienced is commonplace in the U.S. because of the type of dentistry that is practiced. It is a dentistry that treats your mouth as if it were separate from the whole of you, and as a result, ignores obvious connections between your mouth and your body, mind and emotions.

Mercury, an elemental heavy metal, is a neurotoxic poison. Yet a licensed dentist had put this toxic substance in my mouth as a child, and as an adult another dentist had drilled that mercury with a high-speed metal drill – as if it were safe to do so, when it is clearly not safe! Inhalation of, ingestion of and dermal exposure to mercury can cause central nervous system toxicity that can include tremors, memory loss, insomnia, headaches, neuromuscular pain, and cognitive and motor dysfunction. Our liver and kidneys filter toxic substances from our blood, and so mercury can collect in these organs. As a heavy metal, mercury is challenging to detoxify and excrete from the body. It tends to stay in the body if not bound by a binding substance such as silica, chlorella, dimercaptosuccinic acid (DMSA) or dimercapto-propane sulfonate (DMPS) to help the body purge it through the liver/colon or kidneys/bladder. At that time in my life however, I knew nothing about mercury poisoning or mercury detoxification. What happened to me felt like getting blindsided by a crashing wave.

Suddenly, my brain was in a fog. I found myself depressed and anxious and feeling lost. I developed hypothyroid, my kidneys were stressed, and my adrenal glands were exhausted, meaning I was chronically fatigued, reactive and motivated by stress. I often wondered, *what happened?*

At the end of what felt like a long downward spiral, I landed in a hospital having emergency surgery for an ovarian tumor. Having survived the ordeal, I instinctively decided to move from Pittsburgh to Santa Monica, California in search of a new kind of holistic medicine that could help me recover better mindbody health. Fortunately, I found what I was looking for!

One day a new client came into my somatic therapy office with an audio recorder asking if he could record our session, explaining that he had short-term memory problems because of mercury poisoning from mercury amalgam dental fillings. I listened to his story intently, realizing what he was describing had happened to me. He referred me to a monthly informational presentation by Dr. Hans Gruenn, an integrative physician, and Dr. James Rota, a systemic dentist, whose offices in West LA were just a ten-minute drive from me. Thus began a healing journey that would last a decade. Finally, I was getting the answers to the questions I was searching for. During that time, I was blessed to work with multiple oral-systemic dentists to safely remove the mercury amalgam fillings from my teeth, help my body detoxify mercury from my organs with chelating agents, and reestablish better functional alignment in my jaw and bite.

This healing journey in my life provided many opportunities to talk to some remarkable holistic dentists, integrative physicians and detoxification experts. We spoke about the problems in my mouth that were affecting the rest of me, and about the principles and standards of oral-systemic dentistry that would return me to better balance and function. For these enlightening educational conversations, I am forever grateful to systemic dentists Dr. James Rota, Dr. Alireza Panahpour, Dr. Lloyd Herman and Dr. Chester Yokoyama in Los Angeles, and to integrative physicians Dr. Hans Gruenn and Dr. Prudence Hall in Santa Monica, as well as detox chemist Dr. Christopher Shade in Colorado. All of these holistic practitioners helped me recover and sustain better mouthbody health. My goal in this book is to share with you key information I learned from my own experiences to save you time, money and stress.

In the chapters that follow, I review 6 common dental problems that can put your overall systemic health at risk. Each chapter is designed to get you informed fast about the problem and its solution. All of the chapters are important because they explain dental problems that are often interconnected. However, by far the most important chapter is Chapter 8, "Daily Mouthbody Self-Care," because as I will show you in this book, *you* are the most important factor in your mouthbody healthcare, starting with what you put in your mouth every day and consume.

Be mindful about the systemic health effects of consuming sugary foods and drinks or consuming too many antibiotics or tolerating chronic infections in your mouth. For example, we know now that pathogenic bacteria in the mouth were found in arterial plaque in the heart valves of patients who had heart attacks or were at high risk of heart attack. This is one example of the mouthbody connection linking your oral health to chronic illnesses. If you need help letting go of emotional attachments to sugary foods and drinks that you are consuming on a daily basis that you know are bad for your mouth and all the rest of you, get my book *FAST THERAPY: A 10-DAY SELF-HEALING PROGRAM FOR MINDBODY CHANGE* to cleanse, restore and jumpstart healthy changes that last.

CHAPTER 1

A New Paradigm of Oral-Systemic Healthcare

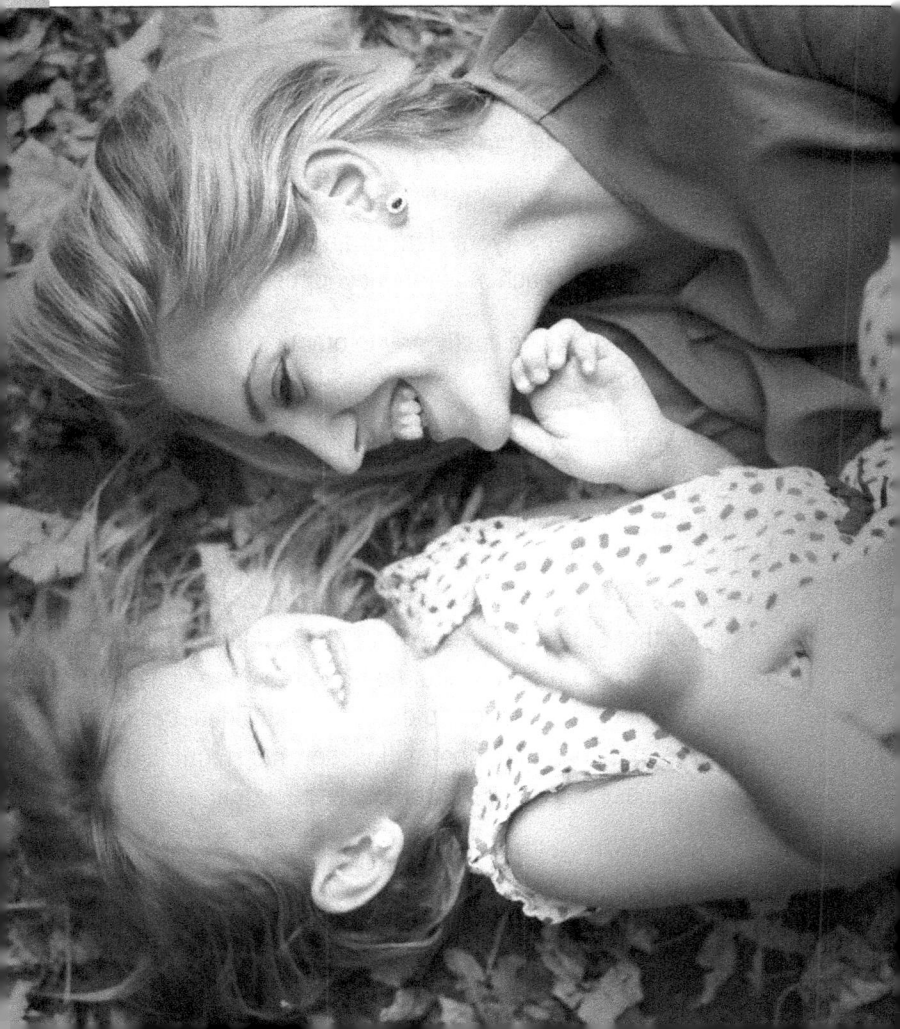

The Problem: Separating Dentistry from General Medicine

Once you understand the connection between your mouth and the rest of your body, it's easy to see the correlations between oral health and a wide range of chronic conditions that are challenging so many people today. The reason is because your mouth isn't separate from your body at all! It's easy to forget that biological and physiological reality in the United States where a profit-driven healthcare system treats and bills your mouth and body separately, requiring you to have two different health insurance plans—one for dentistry to treat your mouth and one for medicine to treat the rest of you.

And typically, the two practitioners who engage those two insurance plans—your dentist and your doctor—don't communicate with each other about your health or treatments.

What an inefficient and costly way to practice dentistry and medicine!

The separation of your mouth from your body might benefit the health insurance industry financially, but it has wreaked havoc on public health. Because most of us have learned to think of our mouths and bodies as separate, we find it easier to accept the invasive and risky treatments conventional dentistry offers us that actually increase our risk of all kinds of chronic conditions. To correct this situation, I want you to understand the mouthbody connection to diabetes, neurodegenerative dementia and so-called mental illnesses, heart, gut, liver and kidney disease, as well as chronic jaw, neck and back pain.

In the chapters that follow, I provide information you need to choose the dentistry and dentist that are right for you. I want you to know there is an alternative dentistry that you can choose that promotes safer practices and supports whole body wellness that is vastly different from the conventional allopathic dentistry of the past. It's a whole different practice with different treatments, materials, protocols and equipment. My goal is to inform you about these differences *before* you sit in a dentist's chair. Because your choice of dentist may be one of the most important decisions you will make to sustain your lifelong health. If you're a parent, you'll also get to make this choice for your children. And if you care for elders, decisions about their mouthbody healthcare may fall to you as well. You get to choose for yourself and your family.

Oral-systemic dentistry that I describe in this book goes by many names—including holistic, integrative, biological or mercury-free. However, whatever name it goes by, you can recognize it by its emphasis on *the mouthbody connection.* Because of its holistic approach, the difference between oral-systemic dentistry and conventional dentistry can look and feel like night and day. Below, I identify the key values that differentiate oral-systemic dentistry from conventional allopathic dentistry. At the end of this book, I provide a list of professional organizations with practitioner directories to help you find a dentist aligned with oral-systemic principles.

5 Key Values of Oral-Systemic Dentistry

These 5 key values are shaping a new paradigm
in dentistry. Search for them and ask for them, and you
will find the dentist and dentistry you are looking for.

1. **Minimally Invasive**

    Oral-systemic dentistry is minimally invasive in its
    treatments, showing a preference for what is safest
    and most beneficial for lifelong mouthbody health. To
    give just one example of this principle, oral-systemic
    dentists will often use air abrasion technology and
    antibacterial ozone gas to treat early-stage cavities
    in tooth enamel. This allows them to avoid drilling
    teeth with a high-speed metal drill—a treatment that
    permanently weakens tooth structure and increases the
    risk of future recurrent decay and tooth fractures. Drilling
    also causes dental trauma. How many people have been
    traumatized in a dentist's chair by the sound and feel
    of a high-speed drill bit drilling away at a tooth inside
    your mouth? Your body instinctively does not like it!

2. **Mercury-free**

    It's a standard practice in conventional dentistry in
    the U.S. to drill cavities and then fill the hole with
    mercury-silver amalgam, and the Food and Drug
    Administration (FDA) allows it. These tooth fillings are
    about 50% mercury. Mercury is a neurotoxic heavy
    metal that is liquid at room temperature, which means
    it is unstable in heat and has the potential to leach into
    your mouthbody—putting your brain, kidneys, liver, gut
    and heart at risk. Sadly, the FDA has for decades failed

to ban this toxic substance from dentistry as Japan and countries in the European Union have done (see the **Minamata Convention on Mercury Treaty** banning industrial and medical uses of mercury which the U.S. has refused to sign.) As a result, in America the burden of choice falls on consumers of dental services to know why they might want to choose a mercury-free dentist over a conventionally trained dentist who uses mercury amalgam for tooth fillings rather than safer, biomimetic materials such as zirconia ceramic. Zirconia ceramic is a non-toxic dental material that mimics the look and strength of natural tooth enamel and is stable at hot temperatures with a melting point over 3000 degrees Fahrenheit compared to mercury's melting point at room temperature. Mercury-free dentistry is also safer for the environment, as wastewater from dental offices carrying mercury has contributed to contaminated water across the United States.

3. **Holistic**
   Systemic dentists are more likely than conventional dentists to talk to you about underlying causes of common dental problems, such as poor nutrition from sugary processed foods, chronic dehydration, imbalances in your oral-gut microbiome, or mouth-breathing and snoring. Systemic dentists will treat your mouth in relation to your other organs, avoiding treatments and procedures that might cause systemic stress on your whole-body health in order to reduce chronic inflammation, chronic infection and chronic toxicity. Such systemic stressors can disrupt the natural health of your immune system and endocrine system, disrupt

your gutbrain health, stress your heart and cardiovascular system, and reduce your ability to detoxify and excrete waste via your liver/colon and kidneys/bladder.

4. **Cost-Effective**

    While oral-systemic dentistry may cost more upfront, it is actually far more cost-effective over time. Conventional dental treatments often contribute to a vicious cycle of drill it, fill it, bill it, followed by crowns, caps, root canals, and eventually implants and dentures – all because these treatments are unnecessarily stressful and invasive and don't address root causes of tooth decay and gum disease. Over decades, they can increase the risk of chronic illnesses the cost of which is hard to even calculate. By investing in systemic dental care today, you can prevent more invasive treatments down the road, saving yourself money and protecting your mouthbody health for years to come.

5. **Informed Consent**

    In my experience, oral-systemic dentists like it when you ask questions about treatments, procedures, materials and equipment. They take the time to educate you and enjoy doing so because they understand that choices you make about your oral health directly impact your overall health. They understand how important it is that you be truly informed before you sit in a dentist's chair and consent to any particular dental treatment. If your dentist can't provide answers to your questions and concerns or doesn't want to take the time to do so, find a systemic dentist who can answer your questions and who values informed consent.

CHAPTER 2

Dental Caries and Tooth Decay

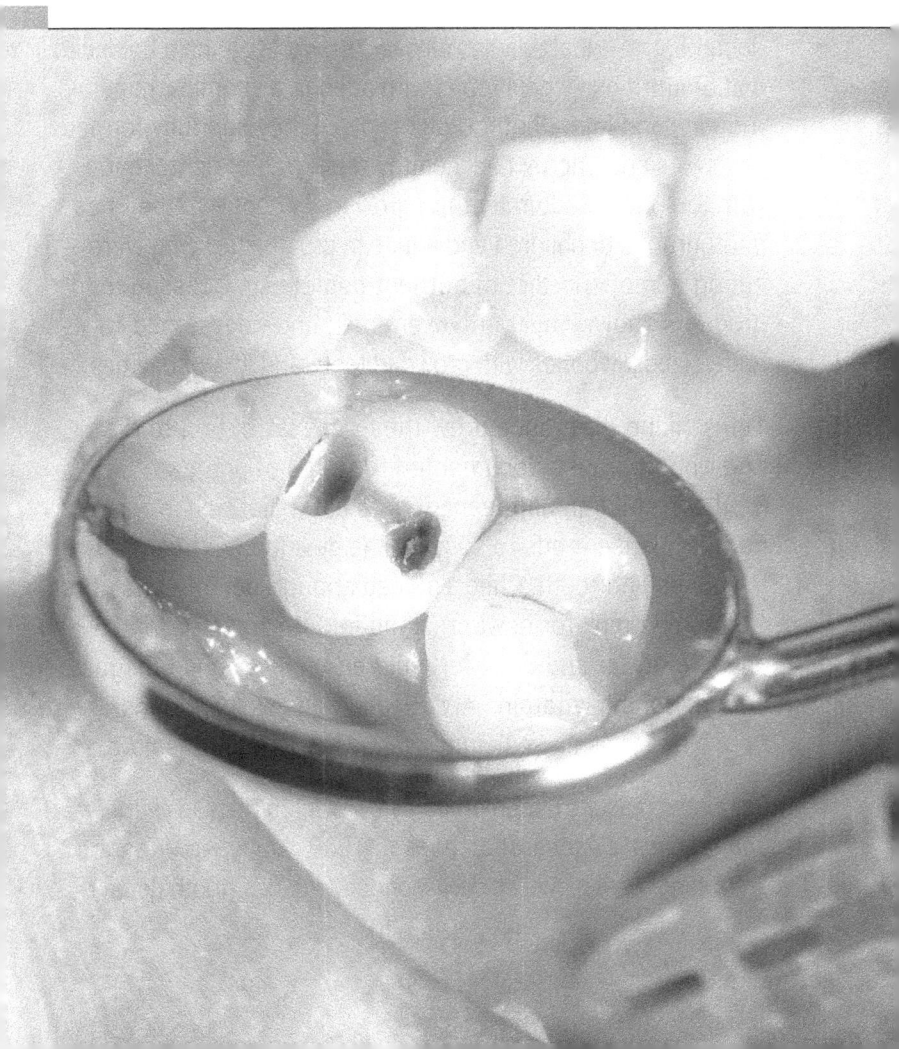

The Problem: A Dental Caries Epidemic

Dr. Weston Price in his now classic book on nutrition and oral health entitled *Nutrition and Physical Degeneration,* first published in 1939, documented in photographs the effects of the modern diet of refined sugar, flour, pasteurized dairy, powdered milk (including baby formula), and canned meats and vegetables on the formation of healthy jaws and teeth. Weston Price and his wife Florence Price traveled extensively, documenting tribal peoples all over the world eating a balanced diet of nutritious whole foods with adequate vitamins, minerals, proteins and fats. Photographs showed they had fully formed jawbones and uncrowded, healthy teeth free of dental caries, with room for wisdom teeth to grow in. In contrast, the Price's photographs of children and adults in urban cities who were eating a "modern" diet of nutrient-depleted, processed food products showed over and over again underdeveloped, undersized jawbones with crowded teeth and lots of cavities.

The striking difference drew the Price's attention to diet. Their photographs documented the need of pregnant mothers, children and teenagers to eat a diet rich in whole, nutrient-dense foods to support the development of healthy jawbones and teeth. Children need enough healthy fats—first from breastmilk for newborns and infants and later fish oil and raw butter and dairy for children—to get good omegas and fat-soluble vitamins A, D, E, and K, as well as foods rich in minerals like calcium, magnesium and potassium.

For all the reasons documented by Dr. Weston Price in *Nutrition and Physical Degeneration* back in 1939, today, Americans are facing a full-blown epidemic of dental caries (tooth decay), including pediatric caries. By 2014, the CDC reported that 42% of children between the ages of 2 and 11 had cavities in their teeth. Imagine the dental trauma for children during those delicate development years! I once had the unpleasant task of accompanying a friend and her young daughter to the dentist to treat *12 cavities in her baby teeth!* Sadly, drilling and filling children's teeth, or worse, giving them baby root canals, will not solve the root cause of the problem. Instead, treating the symptoms of poor nutrition without preventing the cause has only made the problem worse. By 2020, the CDC reported 46% of 2 to 19-year-olds had tooth decay. Not surprisingly, the situation on the other end of the age spectrum is equally alarming, with CDC data showing 13% of adults 65 and older *had lost all their teeth and were wearing dentures.*

Feeding Unhealthy Microbes in Your Mouthbody

Eating inflammatory, nutrient-depleted processed foods—including refined sugar, flour and salt, processed meats, pasteurized low-fat dairy, margarines and trans fats—all feed harmful microbes in your mouth that can travel to different parts of your body. One of these pathogens is candida albicans, a sugar-eating fungus that causes whitish-yellow yeast infections and thrush in the tongue, mouth and throat (also known as oropharyngeal candidiasis). Candida can also populate your intestines and other parts of you—including your vagina, skin, fingernails and toenails—because of the mouthbody connection.

Another common oral pathogen is caries bacteria that eat away at tooth enamel and dentin, creating pockets or cavities that trap food, feeding further bacterial growth. If untreated, the infection can eventually spread from teeth into the jawbone, reducing blood supply to the bone, eating away at it and weakening it over time, and increasing the risk of tooth loss. The inflammation caused by the immune system's response to these chronic infections can speed up jawbone erosion even further.

This vicious cycle explains why so many Americans end up losing their teeth. In "U.S. Population Usage of Dentures from 2012 to 2024," *Statistica* reported that by 2020, over 40 million Americans had lost some or all of their teeth and were wearing dentures. It also projected that by 2024 that number would grow to 42 million Americans. Dentures market analysis published in *SNS Insider Research* in 2024 showed the surging dentures market valued at $1.62 billion in 2023, estimated to nearly double to $3 billion by 2032. That's a lot of money being spent every year to cover up the fact that so many millions of Americans are losing their teeth!

Caries infection in the mouth is considered a chronic infectious disease, and it is transmissible. So please be aware that you can share harmful pathogenic microbes in your mouth with people in your life. Mothers and fathers can pass their oral microbiome to their newborns, infants and children, as can grandparents and other caregivers by sharing food, drinks and utensils, as well as by kissing. So if you are concerned that you might have an infected root canal, infected wisdom tooth cavitation, or recurrent decay from caries infection in your teeth, it's important to address those concerns not only for yourself, but also for the people you love.

Overuse of Antibiotics Makes the Situation Worse

Unfortunately, over-prescribing and over-using antibiotics have made the situation worse, not better, for far too many Americans. Antibiotics are not a simple "fix-it" solution, because antibiotics kill both pathogenic *and* beneficial bacteria at the same time, sometimes causing permanent damage to the mouthbody microbiome. Throwing antibiotics at recurrent dental infections fed by poor nutrition won't solve the problem.

The Solution: A Nutrient-Rich Organic Whole Foods Diet

It helps to find a systemic dentist who understands the mouthbody connection and who practices holistic, biological, minimally-invasive dentistry. However, the best way to prevent rampant tooth decay is by changing your diet to include more nutrient-dense, whole foods that you prepare and cook at home that are easy to digest and absorb. If you've been eating poorly, I understand that changing your diet can be challenging. But if you regularly consume sugary processed foods, you're guaranteed to have more dental problems than you would if you dropped the sugar. By eliminating sugar from your diet and sourcing organic, whole foods rich in bioavailable nutrients, you can reduce the risk of both caries tooth decay as well as yeast infections.

Honestly, too many Americans are eating sugary processed nutrient-depleted foods, suffering weakened immunity as a result, and then popping antibiotics like there's no tomorrow when they get infections in their mouth, gut, lungs or skin. Avoiding overuse of antibiotics is a basic self-care skill we all need to practice in the age of antibiotic-resistant bacteria. Honestly, nothing external can match the natural and acquired immunity that comes from a healthy internal microbiome of beneficial bacteria that keep pathogenic bacteria, viruses and fungi in check.

Ways to Avoid Overusing Antibiotics

Year after year, the Centers for Disease Control (CDC) warns Americans against overusing antibiotics, because overuse has contributed to the rise of antibiotic-resistant strains of bacteria that are making people very, very ill. While antibiotics are sometimes necessary for life-threatening infections, overusing them weakens the body's natural immune defenses and can lead to long-term health issues. Overusing antibiotics early in life can culture the wrong kind of mouth and gut microbiome, leading to early tooth decay and gum disease. For this reason, natural childbirth and breastfeeding are so critical for establishing healthy bacteria in the mouthbody from birth.

If you feel you have already had too many antibiotics in your life, there are several things you can do. Rather than ignore the problem until you get sick and then run to your doctor *demanding* antibiotics for every cold or flu (colds and flu are *viral respiratory infections,* not bacterial, and as such do not respond to antibiotics), instead take responsibility and focus on nurturing your own natural and acquired immunity by changing your diet to support better mouthbody health with prebiotics, probiotics, and nutrient-rich whole foods.

For viral or bacterial infections, consider natural remedies that support stronger immunity before jumping to antibiotics. For example, getting sunshine on your skin and supplementing with Vitamin D as well as eating enough cold pressed virgin olive oil helps our immune response because our liver uses a Vitamin D metabolite, an oleic fatty acid chain (olive oil is the highest source of oleic acid) and a testosterone molecule to metabolize glycoprotein macrophage activating factor (GcMAF), which are the markers for our immune system that help white blood cell macrophages target pathogens for phagocytosis. GcMAF has even been studied as a potential cancer treatment, as some scientists think that GcMAF could combat the enzyme nagalase that cancer cells release to protect themselves. In addition, Vitamin C enhances immune cell function and antibody production, and Vitamin C pairs seamlessly with beta glucans, biologically active polysaccharides sourced from mushrooms. These substances increase immune defense by enhancing macrophages and natural killer cell function. Staying hydrated with immune boosting herbal teas such as ginger, turmeric and green tea as well as proper electrolyte mineral balance and immune-supporting minerals like zinc also support stronger immunity. As does getting more sleep.

In the meantime, ozone therapy is a tool systemic dentists use to treat infections in the mouth while you improve your self-care skills regarding good nutrition. I'm going to tell you about these amazing technologies but if you don't change your diet, more infections will arise and you'll be back in the dentist's chair chasing one tooth cavity after another.

Ozone therapy is truly God's gift to humankind because it's a naturally occurring gas of three oxygen molecules, O3, made naturally when lightning strikes the earth and when sunlight hits the outer layer of our oxygen-rich atmosphere, temporarily splitting oxygen molecules which reform as O3—ozone. O3 is unstable and will eventually return to form more stable O2.

When used therapeutically inside the body via direct IV treatment, ozone gas destroys bacteria, viruses and fungi by splitting their molecules. Ozone gas can be used to treat dental caries, disinfecting the area of tooth enamel without drilling the cavity, which helps keep the tooth structurally intact after treatment. Ozone therapy also includes rinsing the infected area with ozonated water. After 30 minutes or so, ozone returns to O2, releasing the extra oxygen molecule to bind with free radicals in the body, making them less reactive and easier to metabolize and eliminate from the body.

Ozone cannot be patented, which is why most Americans haven't heard of it. It's so incredibly cost-effective no pharmaceutical corporation will ever make any substantial profit from it. It's easily available everywhere you can access medical grade oxygen to put into an ozone generator—a briefcase size device that runs on electricity and is available to the general public for about $3k. Dental ozone therapy can help you treat caries infections in your teeth and so much more. But you have to know about it to ask for it.

In fact, one easy way to determine if you have found a systemic dentist is to ask the dentist if they use ozone therapy in their practice. If the answer is no, you've found a conventionally trained dentist trained to drill it, fill it, and bill it. However, if the answer is yes, you've likely found a systemic dentist who has a variety of alternative treatments for tooth decay that can help you keep your teeth in your mouth for life.

Resources

If you want to learn more about the mouthbody connection, I suggest starting with Weston A. Price's classic book on holistic dentistry *Nutrition and Physical Degeneration*. The book is available in the public domain on Project Gutenberg Australia at **gutenberg.net.au/ebooks02/0200251h.html**. It's also available on the Internet Archive at **archive.org/details/price-nutrition-and-physical-degeneration**. You'll see five pages of illustrations listed at the beginning of the book similar to these that demonstrate the role nutrition plays in oral-systemic health.

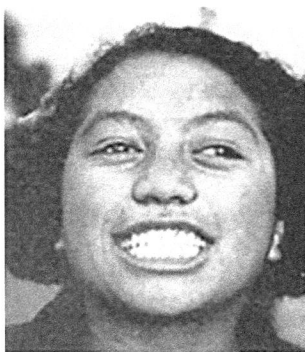

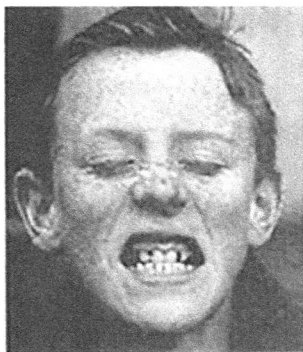

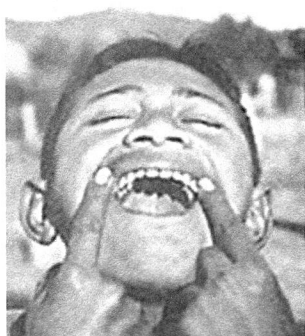

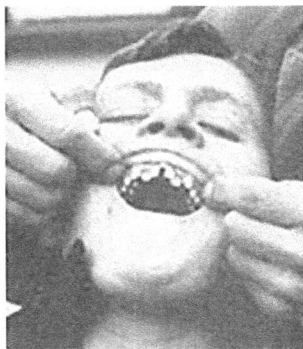

If you like to see dental images including clinical images, go to Google images and search for these keywords to see plenty of examples of topics covered in this chapter. If seeing clinical images makes you stressed, no worries. Skip the images and keep reading to learn how to take action to support better oral-systemic health.

- *Dental caries*

- *Cavities in teeth*

- *Cariogenic biofilm electron microscope*

CHAPTER 3

Gum Disease and Tooth Loss

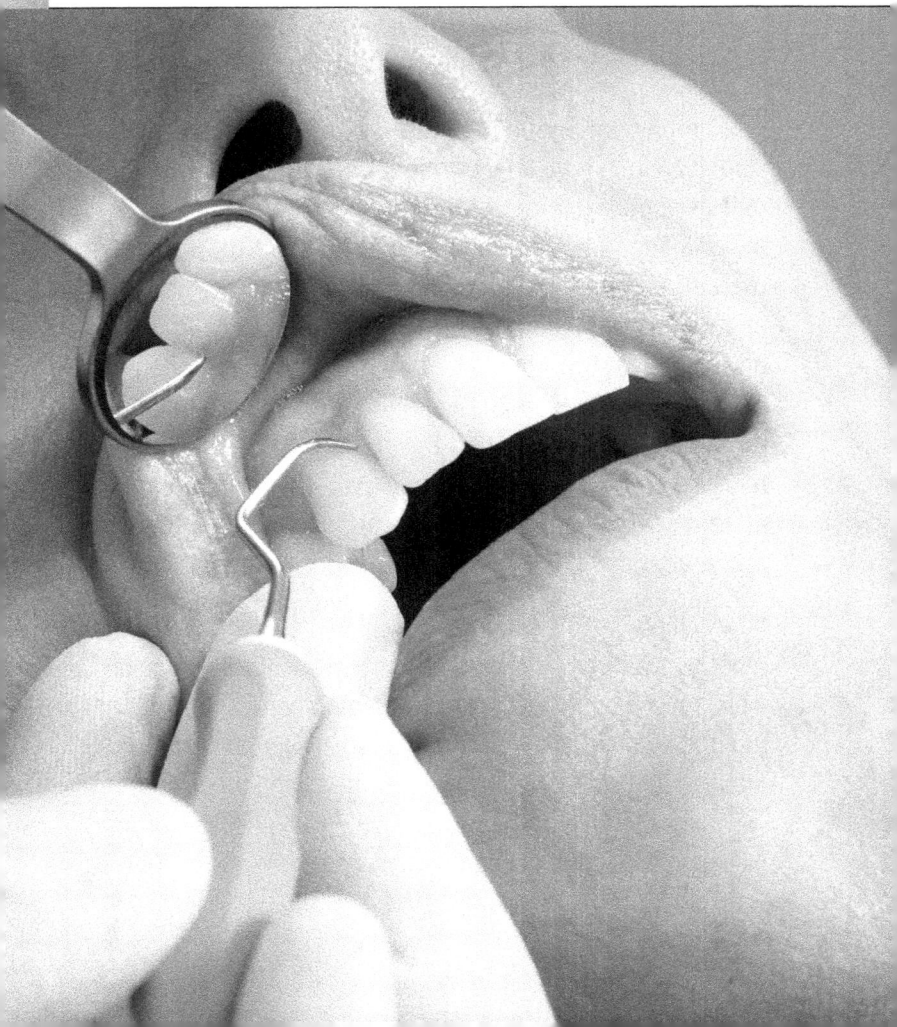

The Problem: Periodontal Disease Linked to Chronic Illnesses

Periodontal disease, also known as gum disease, occurs when harmful bacteria grow unchecked in the gums of the mouth, eating away at the connective tissue around teeth. When periodontal bacteria culture colonies between the gums and teeth, it creates deep pockets of infection. Over time, these pockets of infection can destroy gum tissue and tooth structure leading to bleeding gums and pus, gum recession, loosened teeth, and, if untreated, tooth loss.

The problem of periodontal disease is widespread in the United States, fueled by our poor nutrition from our modern diet of sugary and nutrient-depleted processed foods lacking adequate minerals, good fats and Vitamin D. Old mercury amalgam fillings can contribute to the condition as mercury leaches into the teeth and gums over years and decades. Data published by the American College of Prosthodontists in 2019 estimated about 178 million Americans—more than half the entire U.S. population—are missing at least one tooth, while over 40 million are missing *all their teeth*. Think of the implications of those numbers if oral health is one key marker of overall systemic health.

For example, people suffering from gum disease have 2 to 3 times the risk of heart attack and stroke, because a chronic infection in the mouth increases inflammation throughout the body which can lead to atherosclerosis (hardened arteries) that slows blood flow to the heart and brain. That's why periodontal disease is also linked to higher risk of Alzheimer's disease. In addition, elevated blood sugar from diabetes increases the risk of gum infections and can make infections worse, while periodontal infections can contribute to higher blood sugar levels, creating a vicious cycle that can become degenerative. Left untreated, these infections in your mouth can also lead to higher risk of other chronic systemic conditions including autoimmune disease and cancer.

Periodontal Biofilm

Dentists have known about plaque that forms around teeth and gums for centuries, but in 1978 dentist Bill Costerton identified multiple harmful microbes such as caries bacteria, candida fungus, and periodontal bacteria living together in an aggregate colony under a hard protective casing that he called a *biofilm.* Biofilm plaque protects these pathogenic microbes from detection by the immune system's T-cells and macrophages, and for this reason biofilm is very hard to penetrate and treat.

Understanding the Cause

As discussed in the previous chapter on dental caries, both malnutrition from a poor diet and overuse of antibiotics play major roles in cultivating the wrong kinds of microbes in your gums. Processed, sugar-laden foods promote the growth of harmful microbes, and antibiotics kill off beneficial bacteria, worsening the imbalance over time. Even good oral hygiene won't completely eliminate gum disease if the microbiome in your mouth and gut is unhealthy. Many people realize they have periodontal disease only after the damage is advanced because the bacteria responsible for the infection hide deep in gum pockets invisible to the naked eye.

This silent progression is why gum disease is so common and why it's essential to take proactive steps to prevent and treat it, starting with having regularly scheduled cleanings.

The Solution: Treat the Cause, Not Just the Symptoms

If you have periodontitis—inflammation of the gums—the fastest way to remedy your situation is to address the root cause. Regular dental cleanings are important, including deep pocket cleanings around teeth below the gum line if you need it, but cleanings are only the beginning of the healing process. You also need a good oral-systemic dentist who understands the mouth-body connection who can offer holistic treatments beyond antibiotics. I'll review ozone therapy, food-grade hydrogen peroxide therapy, and red laser light therapy below.

While it may seem logical to buy a toothpaste and/or mouthwash that offers an antibacterial agent, be cautious, because these products can kill beneficial bacteria along with harmful ones, actually making antibiotic-resistant bacteria in your mouth more dominant over time. Remember, gum disease is a systemic issue, not just an oral one, so it requires a holistic approach. Commit to better self-care and lifestyle changes. Even the best dentist can't save your teeth until you take responsibility for your daily mouthbody self-care.

What if gum disease is advanced?

If you have advanced periodontal disease and have been through rounds and rounds of antibiotics trying to save one tooth after another but in the end losing the battle, it may be time to talk to a good systemic dentist about safely and properly removing the teeth and being fitted with dentures. I know that sounds like the least attractive option, but sometimes it is actually the best option for the long term that also provides immediate relief. Often the person feels better mindbody health as soon as the process is complete. The risk of chronic infection and chronic conditions is reduced, pain and suffering resolved, and the need for multiple rounds of antibiotics eliminated. You can also liberate yourself from all those trips to the dentist that can stretch out over years and even decades chasing one fire after another.

If you think this describes your situation, reach out and ask a friend or family member for help. Find someone who can hold your hand through the procedure until you get to the other side and feel better. If you don't know which dentist to go to for a consultation, ask your support person to help you find a good systemic dentist in your area and make an appointment.

Steps to Heal and Prevent Gum Disease

1. **Exercise and Oxygenate:** Regular physical activity helps keep your oxygen levels high, which is important for overall health, including the health of your gums.

2. **Hydrate:** Drink plenty of clean, filtered water daily, and ensure you're getting enough electrolytes, particularly magnesium and potassium, which are crucial for gum and overall health.

3. **Eat Smart:** Prioritize a diet rich in whole, nutrient-dense foods. Avoid processed foods, sugary sodas, and refined carbohydrates, as these promote harmful bacteria in the mouth and gut.

4. **Improve Gut Health:** Since your mouth is the gateway to your digestive system, your gut health and oral health are deeply connected. By improving your gut health, you can positively impact the health of your gums and teeth.

5. **Detox Your Gut and Mouth:** Support your detoxification metabolism and help your body eliminate waste faster from your mouth, intestines, liver and colon because these organs are all connected.

Oxygen Therapies for Periodontal Disease

Oxygen therapies include ozone therapy and hydrogen peroxide therapy. Both are powerful tools for treating gum disease. Both are natural antimicrobial agents that help oxygenate the body, creating an environment where harmful biofilms, like those causing periodontal disease, find it difficult to survive. Biofilms thrive in low-oxygen environments, so introducing oxygen disrupts these harmful colonies.

- **Ozone Therapy:** Ozone gas can be applied directly to infected areas, such as periodontal pockets, to kill bacteria and promote healing. It can also be used in ozonated water for rinsing the mouth.

- **Hydrogen Peroxide Therapy:** Food-grade hydrogen peroxide (H2O2) can be used as a mouth rinse or applied to wounds to disinfect. It can even be administered intravenously to treat systemic infections, though only under medical supervision. It's important to use food-grade hydrogen peroxide (35% solution diluted to 3%) and not the kind found in drugstores.

Red Laser Light Therapy

Red laser light therapy is also known as low-level laser therapy (LLLT) or photobiomodulation. The treatment is easy to apply with a special tool along the gumline to treat periodontal disease by reducing inflammation, promoting tissue regeneration, improving blood circulation in the gums, and reducing bacterial burden in the mouth. It is safe and effective even for pregnant women. The laser can target infected tissue without harming surrounding healthy gums, and it supports tooth bone health in the mouth in a non-invasive manner. Red laser light therapy, like ozone therapy, can be a game changer for treating periodontal gum disease.

Proactive Self-Care

The most effective way to prevent gum disease is by mastering the basics of mouthbody self-care: oxygenate, hydrate, and eat smart. You have the power to prevent periodontal disease and its associated health risks by making these changes.

Additionally, choosing the right dentist—one who treats gum disease holistically and understands the connection between oral health and overall health—should be part of your self-care plan. Holistic treatments like IV vitamin therapy, probiotic therapy, and nutritional therapy can work in tandem with oxygen therapies and red laser light treatments to help restore balance to your mouthbody microbiome.

Natural Oral Remedies

There are many plant-based remedies that can help restore balance to the oral microbiome, as well as binders to help reduce toxic substances in your mouth that can create an imbalance in your oral microbiome and feed periodontal disease.

- **Neem:** Used in Ayurvedic practice for thousands of years, neem can be found in toothpastes or used in oil pulling.

- **Xylitol:** A natural sugar substitute made from the bark of birch trees that kills fungus and harmful bacteria in the mouth without harming beneficial bacteria. You can buy xylitol gum, toothpaste, and mouthwash, or use it in its granulated form sold for baking by putting a spoonful directly in your mouth and swishing for two minutes before spitting it out, repeating the procedure 2-5 times a day.

- **Activated charcoal and silica binders:** Binders like activated charcoal and silica can be used to bind toxic mercury from dental fillings that can contribute to periodontal biofilm, making it easier to remove such toxic substances from the body.

- **Probiotic Toothpastes:** Probiotic toothpaste is a newer development in the treatment of oral dysbiosis. It works by delivering healthy bacteria directly to the mouth, helping to maintain a balanced oral microbiome. While probiotic toothpaste can be a useful tool, it won't be enough if you continue to consume sugary processed foods that feed unhealthy microbes.

Resources

If you like to see dental images including clinical images, go to Google images and search for these keywords to see plenty of examples of topics covered in this chapter. If seeing clinical images makes you stressed, no worries. Skip the images and keep reading to learn how to take action to support better oral-systemic health.

- *Periodontal disease*

- *Periodontal plaque electron microscope*

- *Gum disease and autoimmunity*

- *Red light therapy for gum disease*

CHAPTER 4

Wisdom Teeth Extractions and Osteonecrosis

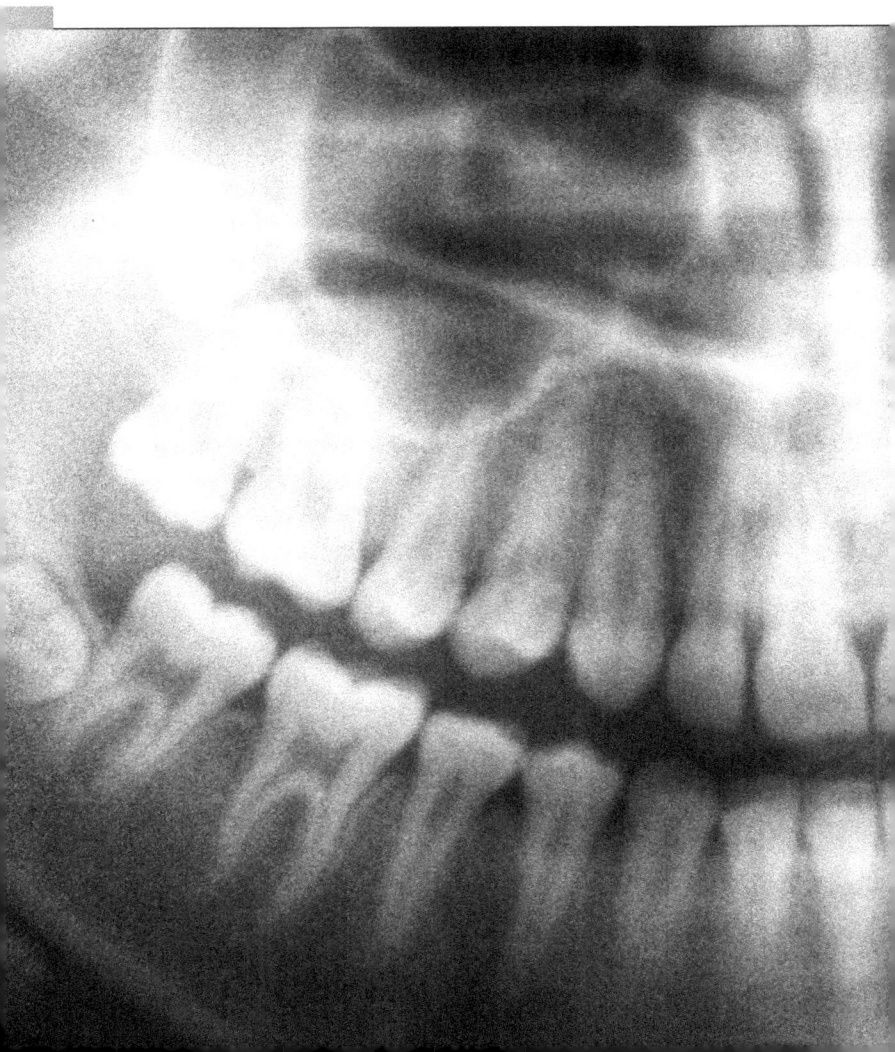

The Problem: Extraction of Wisdom Teeth Is Often Unnecessary

Early wisdom tooth removal, known as prophylactic third-molar extraction, is a standard practice in conventional dentistry today and is approved by the American Dental Association. However, an estimated 80% of early wisdom tooth extractions aren't medically necessary. Nonetheless, the oral surgery has become so common, most young people accept the discomfort and pain of wisdom tooth extraction as a rite of passage to adulthood without realizing the potential long-term health consequences.

While this common dental surgery may be profitable for those dentists who make a living off wisdom tooth extractions, prophylactic third-molar extractions are invasive and can lead to avoidable health risks. One of them is degenerative osteonecrosis (dead bone infected with necrotic bacteria) in wisdom teeth sockets—creating a focal jawbone infection similar to a root canal infection.

Before you agree to amputate a wisdom tooth, make sure the tooth is impacted to the point that it can't emerge through the gumline in functional alignment. When healthy wisdom teeth start to rupture through the gums, of course it feels uncomfortable, just as teething is uncomfortable and irritating for young children. It can be painful while it's happening. However, if the wisdom teeth are not impacted, the pain and discomfort pass after a few weeks as your third molars erupt and grow into proper alignment in your jawbone. This is a dynamic process. Some discomfort and irritation is normal; it doesn't mean that the wisdom tooth needs to be extracted.

The *American Journal of Public Health* published an article in 2007 by systemic dentist Dr. Jay W. Friedman entitled **"The Prophylactic Extraction of Third Molars: A Public Health Hazard,"** raising a red flag about this routine practice in which dentists surgically amputate teenagers' wisdom teeth before they fully develop and rupture through the gums. The invasive practice is so pervasive, an estimated 10 million third molars are extracted from around 5 million young people in the United States *every single year,* generating revenue over $3 billion annually. The problem is—an estimated two-thirds of these invasive surgeries are unnecessary along with the discomfort, pain, bruising and swelling they cause.

Sometimes, these surgeries also cause injury, loss of function, and permanent disability. For example, over 11,000 Americans every year suffer permanent paresthesia after wisdom tooth extraction as a result of nerve injury during the procedure, resulting in numbness of lips, tongue and cheeks. And many young people are left with a chronically infected cavitation deep in the tooth socket in the jawbone.

This serious complication is called Neuralgia-Inducing Cavitational Osteonecrosis (NICO) by some dentists, Fatty Degenerative Osteonecrosis of the Jawbone (FDOJ) by others, or ischemic osteonecrosis by still others. You can find more information by searching any of those names. Swiss Dental Solutions, a leader in the field of treating focal points of inflammation and infection in the jawbone, estimates that 90% of FDOJ are caused by invasive wisdom tooth amputations. The remaining 10% are caused by other tooth amputations or infections resulting from root canal treatments.

In cases of chronic focal infections festering deep inside an empty tooth socket after a tooth extraction, the area in the jawbone around the empty tooth socket becomes soft, mushy and fatty whereas healthy jawbone is hard, solid and firm. Deep infections in the jawbone like this can be difficult to detect because the gums heal over the area quickly, leaving the problem invisible to the naked eye. The condition is associated with chronic pain and nerve damage and higher risk of systemic health conditions such as autoimmune disorders, MS, ALS, and cancer.

For all these reasons, Dr. Friedman in his article in the *American Journal of Public Health* made this blunt statement of caution to consumers of dental services: *"third-molar surgery is a multibillion-dollar industry driven by misinformation and myths."* So be aware that many conventionally trained dentists today still regard prophylactic wisdom tooth extractions as a routine procedure that is as safe as it is profitable—despite all the warnings of serious health risks from oral-systemic dentists.

To make the situation worse, dental insurance providers don't acknowledge NICO, FDOJ or ischemic osteonecrosis. They do not recognize or pay to treat the long-term health consequences associated with the condition. Perhaps because that would mean admitting to the potential harm caused by an invasive procedure that, though often unnecessary, is quite lucrative for the dental industry.

The Solution: Keep Healthy
Wisdom Teeth in Your Mouth

Before you agree to wisdom tooth extractions, whether you are a young adult or you are a parent of a teen, it's essential to determine if the extraction is truly necessary. Take a look at the digital x-rays yourself. Ask for a second opinion if you are unsure. If the teeth are not impacted—meaning they have a clear path to full eruption without jamming into the adjacent molar—consider leaving them alone to grow in naturally.

Prevent Impacted Wisdom Teeth
with Proper Nutrition Early in Life

Whether wisdom teeth will be impacted or not when they grow in depends on good nutrition early in life—starting in utero really, but also in newborn, infant and young childhood years and continuing through adolescence when the skull and jawbone are growing rapidly. Wisdom teeth will be crowded with little room to grow in properly when a teen has a small, underdeveloped jawbone from poor nutrition.

When Wisdom Tooth Extractions Make Sense

Wisdom tooth extraction is a surgical procedure, and like any surgery, it carries risks. But sometimes it is medically necessary. In the estimated 12% of cases where wisdom teeth are truly impacted, alternative treatments—such as removing gum tissue around the tooth to help it erupt—can sometimes solve the problem without removing the tooth itself. However, if surgery is unavoidable, it's crucial to choose an oral surgeon who understands the risks and knows how to minimize them. Teeth are actually structurally similar to fingers and toes. They are surrounded by arteries, veins, lymphatic structures, nerves, and joint cartilage—all held in place by fascia. This makes the amputation of wisdom teeth an invasive procedure that should only be done when absolutely necessary.

How to Identify a Focal Jaw Infection after Wisdom Tooth Extraction

If you've already had your wisdom teeth removed and you suspect a chronic focal infection left behind in your jawbone, pay attention to symptoms like pain or chronic issues on the same side of your body as the extraction site. Problems with your heart, breast, or shoulder can sometimes be linked to an undiagnosed infection in your jaw. Chronic inflammatory conditions can also be involved.

Visit a mouthbody dentist who knows how to read digital x-rays to check for focal infections in empty wisdom tooth sockets. It takes experience to see them as dark shadows in the jawbone that reflect soft mushy areas that should show as solid bone. Getting a thermography of your head, neck and torso can sometimes help by revealing hot spots in the jaw area—a sign of infection.

If you've been diagnosed with a chronic illness and suspect a connection to your past wisdom tooth extractions, consult a dentist experienced in diagnosing and treating chronic focal infections in the jawbone. Be prepared that a conventionally trained dentist may not recognize the condition at all and may tell you your worries are unfounded. Listen to your intuition and seek out a specialist who understands the mouthbody connection and practices oral-systemic dentistry. Play it safe.

Treating a Focal Infection in a Tooth Socket

If an infection is found in an empty wisdom tooth socket in your jaw, the treatment is straightforward but does require surgery. I know that sounds scary, but I've watched the procedure done with two friends and it is actually quite simple. The oral surgeon or general dentist who has training in this type of surgery will inject Novocaine to numb the area. The dentist will then make an incision in the gum tissue to reveal the empty tooth socket. In the first case I witnessed, pus squirted out of the infected cavitation as soon as the incision was made.

The goal of cavitation surgery is to ensure that all infected tissue is thoroughly removed and sterilized so that healthy jawbone can grow back in that area. To this end, the infected area in the jawbone is thoroughly scraped out, cleansed with ozonated water, maybe disinfected with ozone gas, and packed with a plug of platelet rich fibrin (PRF) drawn from your own blood to promote deep and quick healing of the wound from the inside out.

The second treatment I witnessed was quite a surprise to everyone as the surgery revealed a greenish black, dead, underdeveloped wisdom tooth that never erupted fully through the gums. The rotten tooth had been buried in the patient's jawbone for twenty years! The dentist sent the tooth, which smelled horrible, to a lab and the report came back gangrenous (necrotic). In both cases, my friends visibly rejoiced as soon as the pus and infection were removed from their body. Both felt immediate relief of chronic symptoms that included fogginess, anxiety, fatigue, acne around the jaw and neck, stomach distress, adrenal exhaustion, and weakened immunity, as well as inability to conceive and miscarriage.

Resources

If you like to see dental images including clinical images, go to Google images and search for these keywords to see plenty of examples of topics covered in this chapter. If seeing clinical images makes you stressed, no worries. Skip the images and keep reading to learn how to take action to support better oral-systemic health.

- *Impacted wisdom tooth*

- *Healthy wisdom tooth eruption*

- *Neuralgia inducing cavitational necrosis*

CHAPTER 5

Root Canals and Chronic Infections

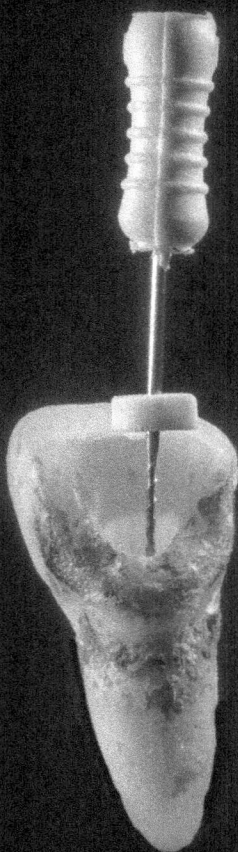

The Problem: Root Canals Are Dead Teeth That Breed Chronic Infection

A root canal is a cosmetic treatment for a dying or dead tooth. First, the top of the tooth is opened and the tooth's root pulp with nerve and blood supply is removed. If the tooth is not already completely dead, now it is. Next, the hollow spaces down the tooth into its roots are filled with gutta percha, a type of rubber-like material, and finally a prosthetic crown is placed on top of the dead tooth. Using this procedure, which is commonplace in cosmetic dentistry, the dead tooth is left in the tooth socket to basically, rot. The patient is left with a root canal tooth that looks cosmetically like a normal healthy tooth on the outside, but inside is actually a breeding ground for pathogenic, anaerobic, necrotic bacteria living in the hundreds of tubules of porous tooth enamel. That chronic focal infection in your mouth will challenge your immune system to deal with the daily exposure, until the infection finds its way into your bloodstream and moves around your body. Obviously, until you remove that infected tissue from your mouth, the focal source of the infection, your immune system will never win this fight. Over time, you become at higher risk of chronic autoimmune conditions and weakened immunity, as well as cancer, including stomach, pancreatic and breast cancer.

The problem with root canal treatment is obvious. Because the tooth is dead, it cultures necrotic bacteria that thrive on dead tissue lacking oxygen. Unlike friendly oxygen-loving bacteria that thrive in a healthy microbiome, anaerobic bacteria living inside our body present a serious challenge for even a healthy immune system. Rounds and rounds of antibiotics cannot change this fundamental situation in your mouth if you have root canals, and the antibiotics can weaken your natural and adaptive immunity even further, or worse, culture antibiotic-resistant strains of bacteria in you that usually eat dead tissue.

When a root canal tooth becomes infected, the infection can spread from the tooth socket into the jawbone, or track along nerves, or spread through arteries, veins and lymphatic vessels to surrounding teeth and beyond into the whole body. Infectious bacteria can move from your mouth to your breasts and heart, for example, or to the brain increasing the risk of stroke. Once clusters of pathogenic bacteria find their way into your bloodstream, they can find their way everywhere, including your pancreas where delicate insulin-making cells and digestive-enzyme-making cells are easily damaged by chronic inflammation as your immune system tries to respond. They can circulate in the bloodstream to be filtered by your kidneys and liver, in turn challenging these core lifegiving organs.

Over time, a chronic focal infection in a root canal tooth can wear down your immune system. It can make you more susceptible to viruses and increasing your risk of chronic inflammatory illnesses, heart disease and stroke, autoimmune disorders, MS, cancer, and other chronic conditions. All because root canal infections affect not only your mouth but your entire body. That's the reality of the mouthbody connection, whether you can see it on Instagram or not.

In spite of all the risks, root canal treatments are big business in the U.S. The American Association of Endodontists reported in its 2024 press kit that over *15 million root canals* are performed *every year* in the U.S., more than 41,000 *every day*—despite the growing evidence that they contribute to a higher risk of a variety of chronic illnesses. The U.S. root canal market was valued at $1.15 billion in 2023, projected to grow to $1.67 billion by 2032. That's a lot of economic pressure to provide root canal treatments whether they are safe for patients or not. And it's a lot of money spent by consumers covering up how many Americans have poor mouthbody health and are losing their teeth at younger and younger ages from poor nutrition.

The Solution: Remove Infected and Dead Teeth from Your Mouth Promptly for Better Systemic Health

Let's be frank. Nobody wants to lose a tooth. However, if your dentist recommends a root canal, you have a choice to make that can impact your overall health for years to come. Many people make the decision to have a root canal under pressure, often when they are in severe pain and desperate for relief. But rushing into a root canal treatment can have consequences. Take your time before making your decision about treatment approach. Get the dentistry you really feel good about, not just in the present moment but long into the future.

Be aware that most oral-systemic dentists will refuse to provide root canal treatments for their patients and don't recommend that patients tolerate them if they already have them. If a tooth gets infected to the point that it can't be saved, these dentists want to extract the tooth immediately rather than prescribe antibiotics and perform a root canal procedure just to keep the dead tooth in your mouth for cosmetic reasons. Instead, they want to get the dead tooth out of your body quickly, without delay. Without delay means as soon as the infected tooth is discovered.

To impress upon you the urgency to remove infected teeth from your mouthbody, I can share a cautionary tale about a dear friend and colleague of mine. She went to her dentist to get her teeth cleaned and was told she had an infected root canal tooth. She had to be told because she didn't feel any pain, because root canal teeth are dead—they have no nerves. However, rather than remove the infected root canal tooth immediately, my friend delayed the extraction for two months because she had planned a trip to see the glaciers in Alaska on a cruise ship. She scheduled her appointment with her dentist for after her return. A few months later, however, my friend began complaining of back pain, and a couple months later was diagnosed with pancreatic cancer and quickly died.

Everyone was in shock because, until she obviously wasn't well, which happened really quickly, she seemed to be in good health. Would she have developed pancreatic cancer even without the root canal infection? Maybe. But we know one precursor to pancreatic cancer is chronic infection. So the risk is real that her infected root canal could have been a contributing factor. There could have been other factors, like high blood sugar. But why risk it? Respond proactively as soon as possible rather than delay, thinking *"oh, it's just my tooth."*

Treating Infected Root Canal Teeth

If you already have a root canal or multiple root canals and you are concerned, search for a systemic dentist who offers alternative treatments that are safer. Your body will thank you for removing an infected root canal in palpable ways that you will sense and feel immediately.

Make sure you choose the right dentist for you. Because you will be offered two completely different options depending on which kind of dentist you choose. If a root canal tooth becomes infected, a conventional dentist or endodontist may prescribe more antibiotics and a second root canal. However, an oral-systemic dentist will prefer to remove the tooth immediately.

If you're concerned for yourself, be proactive. Start a conversation with a systemic dentist about root canals when you get a cleaning. Consult. Gather information and weigh options. Why wait until you notice you have infected pus coming out of the gums around the root canal tooth and you have to rush to the dentist with a dental emergency?

If you already have a root canal, it's understandable that this information may be hard to hear. However, removing the *root of the problem* will free your immune system from a daily fight against a hidden focal infection. After properly removing an infected root canal tooth, people often experience a sense of relief, a boost in energy, a release of stress and a rush of feel-good happy hormones.

Keep in mind that a root canal tooth with a hidden infection deep in the tooth socket can spread infectious bacteria to adjacent tooth sockets where they have access to the roots of nearby healthy teeth. As a result, over time many people are told by their endodontist that they now need additional root canals on neighboring teeth. Throughout this process, often rounds and rounds of antibiotics wear down the immune system even further.

If you're unsure about whether your root canal is causing issues, non-invasive thermography can help detect infections. Infections in the jaw often show up as deep red "hot spots" in thermographic images, making it easier to assess if a root canal tooth is infected.

But My Root Canal Tooth Doesn't Bother Me; I Don't Feel Any Pain

It won't! A tooth that has been given a root canal treatment has no nerve supply or blood supply, so you will never feel pain from a root canal tooth, even if it is becoming infected. Only when the infection spreads into surrounding gums or into surrounding teeth or into the jawbone around the tooth socket or into adjacent nerves will you feel pain and discomfort. If you notice pus around the gum line, imagine that infection deep down in the roots of the tooth where you can't see.

Chronic illness prevention for autoimmunity, multiple sclerosis, cancer, arthritis, heart disease and stroke means reducing your risk of these chronic degenerative conditions by taking action before you become ill. If you have these chronic illnesses in your family history, or you've been given a warning or even a diagnosis by a physician, tell a systemic dentist about your situation and ask them to assess your mouth for any issues that may be contributing to your chronic ill health.

Most systemic integrative physicians and naturopaths are trained to ask you about your dental history when examining you. And many team up with a holistic systemic dentist to whom they make patient referrals. If you need help, ask for help and you'll get it. Just be sure you're asking the right practitioner. Unfortunately, that may not be an endodontist who makes a living off root canal treatments. Just saying. As a consumer, the choice is yours, and that is the greatest power that you have in a consumer culture. It sounds trite and I know I keep saying it, but it's so true: *put your money where your mouth is.* Do what's best for your long-term systemic health.

A Safer Alternative to a Root Canal Treatment: Implants

Nobody wants to lose a tooth. People have bad dreams about losing teeth for a reason. It's traumatic to lose a tooth. However, properly removing an infected, dying or dead tooth and replacing it with an implant (a post that is screwed into the jawbone on which to attach a prosthetic crown) is safer than having a root canal treatment and leaving the compromised tooth in your mouth, for the reasons I have explained in this chapter. Your choice to have a root canal treatment or to remove the tooth and have an implant is one of the most important choices you can make for your lifelong oral-systemic health. However, the implant procedure does require that you have enough healthy jawbone in that area to anchor the implant post into. While a graft of autogenous jawbone (harvested from your own jaw) or donated cadaver bone can be used to create more stability for the implant, too much loss of jawbone around the tooth socket of an infected tooth is a problem. For this reason, time is of the essence. The longer you tolerate living with an infected tooth in your mouth, including an infected root canal tooth, the more bone loss you may suffer, making it more difficult to undergo a successful implant procedure.

Many people delay going to the dentist because there may be pain involved or there may be the memory of past dental trauma. However, going to an oral-systemic dentist sooner than later is always the better option if you are dealing with an infection in your mouth. Infectious bacteria can spread from your mouth to different parts of your body, and can even cause heart attack or stroke. Chronic infections hidden in your mouth put stress on your immune system and can trigger a runaway inflammatory response that over time can become an autoimmune condition. If you need help making an appointment or physically getting to your dentist's office for an exam and consultation, ask for help from a family member or friend who can be your support person to nudge you through your process. Sometimes someone needs to pick up the phone for you and make that appointment, or drive you to the dentist's office. Whatever it takes. If you're having trouble, verbalize what you need and ask for help. That will get the ball rolling.

There are two preferred dental materials used for implant posts: titanium and zirconia ceramic. You will have a choice. Zirconia is more expensive to manufacture than titanium, making zirconia ceramic implants more expensive. Many oral-systemic dentists prefer zirconia ceramic implants over titanium because titanium is a metal, and while it has a long and proven record of being durable and biocompatible, it can turn the gum tissue around the implant grey in color over time. This discoloration makes zirconia ceramic posts preferable for many dentists and their patients, because zirconia does not discolor the gums. Zirconia ceramic is a biomimetic material that is well-tolerated by the body. It looks like natural tooth enamel, is strong, durable, and non-allergenic. Both zirconia ceramic and titanium are long-lasting—from 10 to 15 years, 25 years, even a lifetime if you maintain good oral-systemic health including proper nutrition with adequate calcium, magnesium, zinc, Vitamin D, good healthy fats and enough daily walking for oxygenation of healthy gums and weight-bearing exercise to maintain healthy bone repair and growth. Your teeth are bones, so what's good for your teeth is also good for the rest of your skeleton.

Most systemic dentists who specialize in implants offer the option of general anesthesia during implant procedures which can reduce the stress the patient may experience from the surgery. You will have a choice about whether you want to use a local anesthesia and be awake and actively engaged in the procedure or anesthetized and 'asleep' for it.

The process of placing an implant has several steps. First, the dentist has to properly amputate the dead or dying tooth and thoroughly clean out the empty tooth socket of any debris, tooth ligaments or tooth fragments. Next, the area deep in the jawbone needs to be sterilized with red laser light, and rinsed with ozonated water to reduce the risk of infection. You will have a choice whether you want your oral surgeon to anchor the titanium or zirconia ceramic post (to which a zirconia crown is later attached) into your jawbone immediately after the tooth amputation, or wait until that area completely heals, which usually takes about 90 days, and then anchor the post of the implant into your jawbone later in a separate procedure. The choice is between having two surgical procedures or one. I've experienced both methods and I prefer having both the tooth extraction and the implant insertion done at the same time because the total time it takes to heal completely is faster.

If the condition in the tooth that caused it to become infected ended up compromising tissue in the jawbone, causing bone loss, your dentist may add bone graft to that area. You will have to choose between a graft of your own bone or a graft of donor bone. To fill the empty tooth socket, usually Platelet-Rich Fibrin (PRF) is used to pack the area in order to enhance healing and regeneration deep in the tooth socket. PRF is a natural autologous substance extracted from your own blood and spun in a centrifuge to allow platelets and growth factors to concentrate in a fibrin clot. PRF can also be mixed with calcium. About 90 days after the implant is successfully anchored into the jawbone and the area has healed properly without infection, a zirconia crown is place permanently onto the implant post which looks like the original tooth.

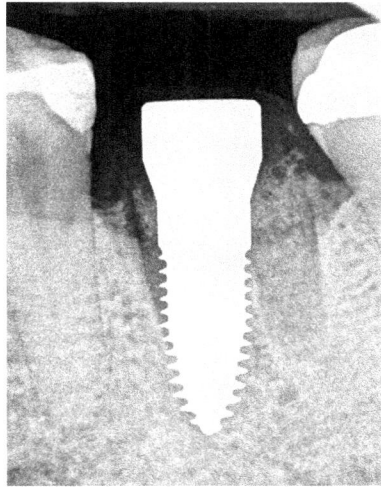

Implants should be cared for the same as natural teeth, with flossing, brushing, using an oral water irrigator, abundant sunshine for Vitamin D metabolism, a healthy balanced diet of organic whole foods, in addition to plenty of healthy exercise. Ultimately, the duration of any implant depends on the patient's self-care and the ability to reverse a pattern of tooth loss.

Resources

If you like to see dental images including clinical images, go to Google images and search for these keywords to see plenty of examples of topics covered in this chapter. If seeing clinical images makes you stressed, no worries. Skip the images and keep reading to learn how to take action to support better oral-systemic health.

- *Infected root canal*

- *Thermography of infected root canal tooth*

- *Zirconia ceramic implant*

CHAPTER 6

Amalgam Dental Fillings and Mercury Toxicity

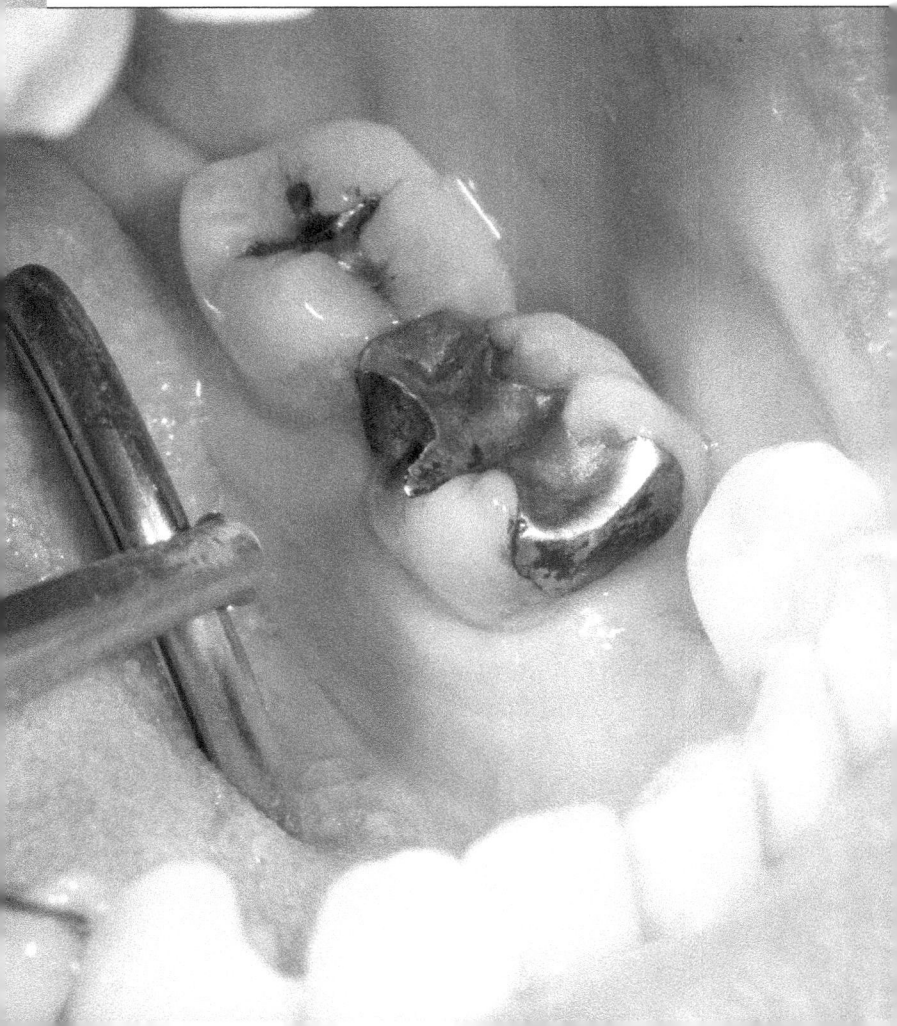

The Problem: Putting Mercury in Your Mouth is Risky Business

Mercury-silver amalgam (about 50% mercury) is one of the cheapest dental materials available; however, it comes with significant risks. Mercury is a potent neurotoxin—even a tiny amount is poisonous to nerves, and a little bit can contaminate an entire lake. Some forms of mercury like methylmercury and mercury chloride are classified as possible carcinogens. In addition, mercury is a heavy metal that is liquid at room temperature, meaning it is unstable as a dental material when exposed to heat, causing leaching, and it expands and contracts with heat and cold. Over time, this expansion and contraction causes margins around the fillings that lead to recurrent decay, more drilling and filling, and eventually to tooth fractures which pave the way for caps and crowns and eventual tooth loss. Under high heat conditions such as high-speed drilling, the mercury in amalgam dental fillings vaporizes and can be breathed, entering the bloodstream through the lungs and quickly dispersing everywhere into the body, including the brain, liver and kidneys.

For all these reasons, the World Health Organization (WHO) considers mercury to be one of the top ten toxic substances of major public health concern. According to the Environmental Protection Agency's (EPA) report "Health Effects of Exposure to Mercury" (2024), chronic mercury poisoning's insidious onset and nonspecific signs and symptoms are easily misdiagnosed as Parkinson's disease, dementia, metabolic encephalopathy, schizophrenia, epilepsy, among many other chronic conditions such as chronic fatigue, anxiety, depression, panic attacks, learning disorders, and cognitive and memory loss. According to a WHO Fact Sheet, mercury has toxic effects on the nervous, digestive, immune and detoxification systems, and on the brain, lungs, heart, kidneys, liver, bowels, skin and eyes. Mothers can pass mercury to their vulnerable unborn babies through their placenta, making it a potential risk factor for autism spectrum disorders and developmental delays in children.

One could imagine that no medical professional in their right mind would expose their patients and themselves and their dental hygienists to toxic mercury. Yet for more than a century, dentists in the U.S. have been doing just that when they fill their patients' cavities with mercury amalgam or drill amalgam fillings to place larger fillings or crowns. Given all these risks, it's natural to wonder why this questionable practice ever became the norm in dentistry.

The answer has to do with our addiction to burning coal to generate electricity. Mercury is naturally found in coal, and so when coal is mined, mercury is mined, and when coal is combusted for energy, mercury is also combusted. This process releases toxic mercury vapor along with carbon dioxide, sulfur dioxide, nitrogen oxide, and carbon monoxide into the atmosphere, some of which comes back down to earth in acid rain that has poisoned forests and waterways across the country. Mining and burning coal for energy is dirty business.

The coal industry has come up with ingenious ways to dispose of its toxic mercury waste, since the EPA prohibits the coal industry from dumping toxic mercury directly into the environment. Instead, the mining industry creates commercial markets to sell its toxic mercury waste to. Remember compact fluorescent light bulbs that were marketed as a "green" solution to incandescent light bulbs? The mercury in those CFL bulbs was so toxic we were told not to throw the bulbs in the trash. How many people knew they were supposed to drive old bulbs to a hazardous waste collection site for safe disposal? Or knew that if they dropped and broke a CFL bulb in their home, business or hotel room, they were supposed to evacuate and call a local hazmat crew for cleanup! Honestly, how many Americans buying and handling CFL bulbs understood these risks?

For decades mercury was also sold as a preservative in vaccines given to vulnerable children, creating another market for mercury. While mercury has been eliminated from childhood vaccines in the U.S. since 2001, some flu vaccines marketed to Americans every flu season still contain the mercury-laced preservative Thimerosal.

In a similar way, the coal mining industry has treated dentistry as an acceptable marketplace for toxic mercury in the form of mercury-silver amalgam used for dental fillings, arguing that combining mercury with silver and a few other metals into an amalgam makes the mercury stable. Any honest dentist who has been practicing for twenty years will tell you that's untrue! However, if profit is your primary goal, it seems any market will do whether it's safe for the public health or not. As a result of this unregulated market logic, today, an estimated 100 million Americans have mercury amalgam fillings in their mouths.

I know this information can be disheartening to people who have mercury fillings in their teeth right now. To say we need better environmental stewardship and regulation from the FDA at this critical moment in our public health history is an understatement. At the time I wrote this book, mercury amalgam dental fillings are still used in the U.S. and their application is still taught in dental schools. Most dental insurance policies in the U.S. cover cheaper mercury amalgam dental fillings but not biomimetic zirconia ceramic fillings or other safer alternatives that cost more.

What can you do? As a consumer living in a consumer culture, you can put your money where your mouth is and find a mercury-free dentist! Ask for one and you'll find one because they're everywhere. As I said in the Introduction, the choice is yours, but you have to choose *before* you sit down in a dentist's chair.

The Safer Solution: Mercury-Free Dentistry

Mercury-free dentistry is systemic, therefore a minimally-invasive approach is used for treating caries infections of tooth enamel that are often signs of sugar consumption, essential nutrient deficiencies and gut-mouth microbiome imbalances. For example, to treat a caries tooth infection caught early, a systemic mercury-free dentist may use air abrasion instead of drilling to remove the decayed area of tooth enamel without damaging any more of the tooth's natural structure. Air abrasion can be followed by an application of ozone gas to kill the pathogenic caries bacteria, rinsed with ozonated water, and followed by an application of zirconia ceramic or other biomimetic material to fill the cavity. As you read in Chapter One, zirconia ceramic is a dental material that looks naturally like teeth, and is safer, stronger, more durable and more stable because it has a melting point of over 3,365 degrees Fahrenheit—meaning it does not expand and contract.

Safe Removal of Mercury Fillings

If you have mercury amalgam fillings in your teeth, and you decide to remove them from your mouthbody, choose a dentist who runs a mercury-free practice. Mercury-free dentists know how to remove mercury amalgam fillings safely by following a strict safety protocol, such as the International Academy of Oral Medicine and Toxicology's (IAOMT) SMART protocol. SMART stands for **Safe Mercury Amalgam Removal Technique**. Read about the SMART protocol and study it so that you know what to ask for when choosing a dentist to help you. If you ask your dentist about their mercury filling removal safety protocol, and they don't know what you're talking about, find a mercury-free dentist who does by using the directory links in the last chapter of this book. Start with the **IAOMT directory** to find a mercury-free dentist.

The SMART protocol requires taking activated charcoal before the procedure, wearing protective gear for eyes and face, wearing a nasal oxygen mask to prevent breathing mercury vapor, ventilation in the room, a Horton 'elephant trunk' vacuum to capture mercury vapor around the mouth area, and a dental dam to prevent swallowing mercury particulate. If your dentist looks like Darth Vadar during the procedure, you know you're in good hands.

Self-Care If You Have Mercury Fillings in Your Mouth

If you have amalgam fillings in your teeth, you can help yourself by reducing your environmental mercury exposure by avoiding fish high in mercury such as tuna and swordfish, preferring smaller fish such as mackerel, sardines and trout. You can also chew chlorella or activated charcoal in the morning, swishing it for a few minutes before spitting it out (somewhere other than your sink as it may stop it up). You can also be mindful to drink room-temperature liquids and wait for cooked food to come to a warm temperature rather than eating foods that are hot.

Avoid grinding your teeth. An hour before bed, turn off your smartphone and TV and let your eyes reset onto the horizon into a relaxed state. Your eyes muscles and jaw muscles are connected; if your eyes are tense your jaw will be too. Take some time to close your eyes, massage your jaw muscles, stretch your neck and stretch open your mouth to relieve stress and tension and assist relaxation. Use proper supportive pillows at night, or no pillow at all, to properly align your skull including your jaw and your neck to keep them relaxed but supported while you sleep.

If a moment in time comes when you choose to remove mercury amalgam fillings from your mouthbody, there's a lot you can do to prepare. Before, during and after mercury filling removal, it's important to support your body's detoxification organs—the liver/colon and kidneys/bladder—by cleansing them of waste. After the fillings are removed, consider a full heavy metal detox under the guidance of a practitioner who specializes in it. During and after the removal, I recommend the **mercury detox products** offered by Dr. Christopher Shade at **QuicksilverScientific.com.** With proper preparation, you can experience a quick recovery after and a healing rebound into higher function and better holistic health.

If you've decided to remove mercury amalgam from your mouth, and you have an attachment to sugar, it's time to break up! Whether it's spoonfuls of sugar in your coffee in the morning, or a glass or two of wine every evening, or soda in the afternoon, or sweet treats between meals, drinking and eating too much sugar puts you at higher risk of chronic dental issues that stress your teeth and gums and compromise your overall health. For this reason, if you want to prevent cavities caused by caries bacteria in your mouth eating away at your tooth enamel, the first thing to do is eliminate refined sugar from your diet. Just read the labels and decline to put it in your mouth. If you drink a lot, get sober. Wine and other forms of alcohol are sugar!

Drink plenty of clean alkaline filtered or spring water throughout the day and cook organic whole foods grown in mineral-rich soils that are nutrient dense and easy to digest. You'll need enough minerals in the proper ratio (twice as much calcium as magnesium, for example, but you need them together) and enough Vitamin D3 (from sun on your skin or raw dairy) with Vitamin K (dark leafy greens) to get calcium into your bones and teeth. You also need enough good fats and enough glycine (an amino acid protein) to build and repair fascial tissue connecting your teeth to your jawbone and gums. Supplement if you need to but give your mouthbody what it needs to be well.

Dealing with Chronic Illnesses

Many integrative doctors recommend that patients with chronic illnesses such as cancer, diabetes, epilepsy, MS, Parkinson's or Alzheimer's consult with a holistic, oral-systemic dentist if they have dental issues. Because many do. Toxic dental materials, or chronic infections in the jaw or gums that we'll discuss in coming chapters, can affect your whole-body, systemic mindbody health in a variety of ways. If there's an issue, have your doctor and dentist talk to each other so they can team up. If they are both systemic practitioners who understand the mouthbody connection, they'll understand why and will be happy you asked.

Resources

If you want more information on mercury fillings, I recommend watching the documentary ***Mercury Undercover*** for a quick history and overview. if you want to get an assessment of your mercury level, Dr. Christopher Shade whom I mentioned earlier, developed the **Mercury Tri-Test** that set a new industry standard for assessing mercury levels in the body. You can also find additional educational resources on dental mercury at the **International Association of Oral Medicine and Toxicology**.

If you like to see dental images including clinical images, go to Google images and search the keywords below to see plenty of examples of topics covered in this chapter. If seeing clinical images makes you stressed, no worries. Skip the images and keep reading to learn how to take action to support better oral-systemic health.

* *Mercury amalgam fillings*

* *Zirconia fillings*

* *Dental air abrasion*

* *Dental ozone therapy*

* *Mercury Tri-test*

CHAPTER 7

Tmj, Misaligned Bite and Scoliosis

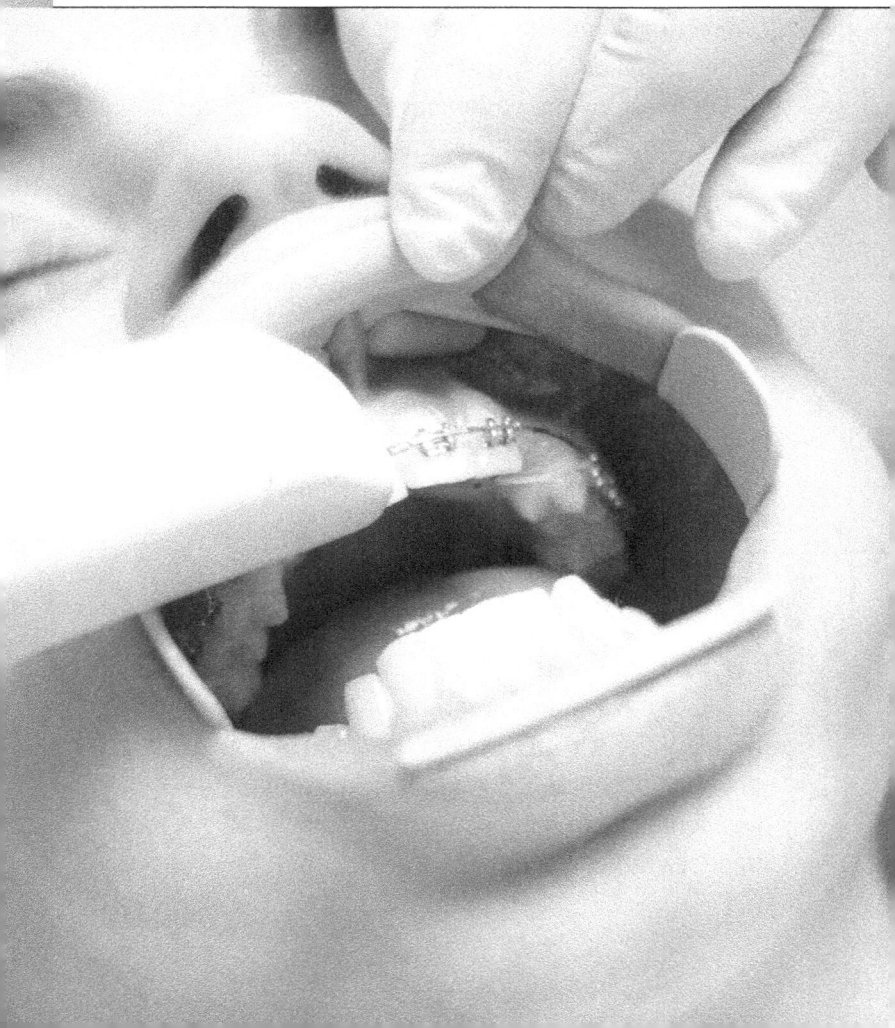

The Problem: Misaligned Teeth and Jaws Affect Whole Body Alignment

The alignment of your teeth and jaw coordinates with your skull and neck for chewing and swallowing, coordinates with your eyes for seeing, and coordinates with your pelvic and sacral alignment affecting your hips, knees and feet when walking and moving. Your skull includes 8 cranial bones and 14 facial bones—all with suture lines connecting them with cartilage, ligaments and fascia. While cranial bones "breathe" and move slightly at the suture lines, the only truly moveable bone in your skull is your mandible, or jawbone. Proper functional mouthbody alignment allows you to chew, swallow, yawn, talk, emote, see, walk and move about without discomfort or pain.

However, even a seemingly slight misalignment in your bite—from a dental filling, cap, crown or implant that's set too high or too low, or from crowded teeth or missing teeth— can cause disharmony in your mouthbody that sends stress lines through your skull and spine affecting your entire skeleton. A misaligned bite can cause headaches, difficulty chewing, a painful walking gait, neck-shoulder-back pain, as well as snoring and sleep apnea. Misalignment in your jaw can even disrupt normal organ and gland function.

If you are challenged by temporomandibular joint pain (TMJ), or have trouble chewing or suffer chronic neck pain, look for a structural dentist who understands the mouthbody connection to check your bite for any misalignment. To find out if a dentist understands and practices structural dentistry, ask them if they use tools

like *Anomalous Medical 3D Dental Anatomy Simulation.*
This digital resource provides more detailed information
about bite alignment than standard x-rays and can help
ensure that any dental work doesn't inadvertently cause
or worsen structural misalignment. If your teeth are
causing your jaw to be misaligned, structural dentistry
can help you return more optimal balance and function
that feels better when you eat meals, talk, sleep at night,
wake up in the morning, and set sail into your day.

If you find yourself grinding your teeth while sitting at the
computer, your jaw-pelvis axis is telling you it's time to
stand up and take a walk! If you're grinding your teeth
at night, it's the same message! You're sitting too much
during the day and not walking and exercising enough
in your life. When you're not chewing food, what your
mouthbody really wants is some alkalinizing hydration
and brisk movement of your legs, as your psoas muscles
and jaw muscles are connected—if you're walking and
running, you're not chewing and eating, and if you're
chewing and eating, you shouldn't be walking or running!
Spare your teeth the wear and tear and give yourself what
you really want and need. Exercise prevents snacking
on sweet comfort foods and overeating as well.

Orthodontics and Scoliosis

Many American children grow underdeveloped jawbones
as a result of their diet of nutrient-depleted processed
foods causing crowded teeth, overbites, underb tes and
misaligned jaws. Overuse of baby pacifiers in infants

is also a contributing factor, especially if you send a baby to bed with a pacifier in its mouth to fall asleep. Sucking a pacifier for years during rapid development of a growing skeleton can alter the shape of the soft palate, causing misalignment in the upper teeth and deviating the natural bite. Orthodontics is commonly used with children and teens to treat misaligned teeth, deviated jaw and/or deviated palate to bring better alignment to the teeth and mouth and improve the bite. The best age to start that correction is around age 6.

However, one has to be very careful with orthodontic interventions because they can cover over the symptoms of poor nutrition, causing people to miss opportunities to make healthy changes in their diet. After treatment, children and teens may look like they have a fully formed healthy mouth with straight uncrowded teeth, when actually they do not. Pregnant and nursing women want to be especially mindful about dietary choices because mothers are prone to lose teeth if they lack the nutrients to feed both themselves and their child.

Another reason to be mindful about orthodontics is because when you change the alignment of the teeth and bite with braces or with a palate expander, you can affect the alignment of the entire spine in a way that causes deviation of the spine, or *scoliosis*. The connection between orthodontic appliances and scoliosis has been well documented, much to the credit of John Upledger of the **Upledger Institute,** who shared his findings working with **young patients with scoliosis** as a cranial-sacral osteopath. In case after case in his practice, he noticed that the sudden onset of scoliotic deviation of the spine followed the application of orthodontic appliances on the teeth, and that the deviation of the spine typically remitted when the braces were removed.

The growing realization that orthodontics in the mouth is connected to deviation in the spine has led to innovations in orthodontic appliances that are designed to adjust the bite. Many appliances are removable and can be worn only at night or for so many hours a day. Such adaptations have made orthodontic treatments more holistic and less invasive.

The Solution: Choose a Dentist Trained in Structural Dentistry

If you're experiencing problems like TMJ, headaches, or chronic neck/shoulder/back pain and you suspect a misaligned bite, search for a holistic dentist who specializes in structural dentistry. Structural dentists are meticulous about ensuring that any dental work—whether fillings, caps, crowns or implants—doesn't throw off your bite. They can also create custom dental appliances designed to realign your bite over a period of time if it is misaligned to the point that it reduces function.

If you feel you need orthodontic help to optimize your bite and bring better alignment to your teeth, or you think your child needs orthodontics, take your time choosing a structural dentist who understands the risks, can mitigate stress on the spine, and monitor any changes to make appropriate adjustments to prevent spinal deviation. If the misalignment in your teeth is cosmetic rather than functional, you might want to think twice before choosing orthodontic treatments.

Erin Myers, author of *I Have Scoliosis: Now What?* is a Pilates instructor supporting the scoliosis community through **_Spiral Spine Scoliosis Care_**, an online hub for those with scoliosis. Myers recommends caution regarding orthodontic interventions, favoring the needs of the spine over the teeth in cases of malocclusion. She shares, *"In my case, where scoliosis wasn't present but malocclusion was, I had a deviated jaw but a straight spine. I wonder what would've happened to my straight spine if I had left my deviated jaw where it was. After my orthodontic work, I had a straight jaw and a deviated spine. If research shows that there's a positive correlation between the alignment of the jaw and the spine, realizing there is a correlation between orthodontics and scoliosis isn't hard to fathom."*

It's important that parents understand the connection between orthodontic braces and appliances and scoliosis, because in the conventional allopathic healthcare system we have in the U.S., invasive surgery is offered young patients who develop severe scoliosis. Metal rods are placed along the spine to guide it to grow straight. From a holistic, oral-systemic perspective, this is a unfortunate path to go down. It's treating an invasive treatment's adverse effect with an even more invasive treatment still. Think of the stress these treatments place on young people who may not understand what is happening to them, because they are unaware of the mouthbody connection.

It can be traumatizing. I had a 19-year-old client once who came to me having had a suicide attempt at 13, and a longtime struggle with depression. On intake, I asked her about her dental history, and saw the light bulb go off for her when she realized the braces on her teeth preceded not only the scoliosis in her spine but also the suicide attempt that followed the painful spine surgery used to treat her severe scoliosis. I texted her several links to articles to read, and she looked so relieved to realize what happened to her wasn't *"all in her head."* Once she understood what happened to her, she was able to work with what she has and get on with living her life. But she also knew if she had children one day she would take a less invasive approach to straightening their teeth and correcting bite issues.

Use a Team Approach to Optimize Results

Structural dentists are likely to refer you to a chiropractor, cranial-sacral practitioner, or osteopath to help your whole body adjust to dental treatments in order to maintain proper alignment. The team approach can provide significant relief from chronic pain and discomfort and speed up the results, promoting better balance throughout your entire body, allowing more ease and function while chewing, smiling, talking, walking and exercising – even thinking and feeling. Because if your jaw is out of alignment, your skull and neck will be out of alignment, and so on down the line to your pelvis and feet. From an oral-systemic point of view, if your bite is out of alignment, that means *you* are out of alignment! And as a result, you might find yourself feeling cloudy-headed, irritable, anxious, depressed and 'out of balance' in your moods, emotions and thoughts. These symptoms are all expressions of the mouthbody connection.

Teaming up with a skilled chiropractor or cranial-sacral osteopath during and after dental work can help you recover your natural bite and gait faster and maintain them longer while restoring better balance in your body from your eyes down to your toes. It's a dynamic process and takes some time, though relief is often immediate. I work with a cranial-sacral osteopath on the west side of L.A. on a regular basis to help myself maintain balanced alignment for optimal function and minimal discomfort. It's a work in progress, as I've had a lot of dental trauma that has left me with two missing teeth and an imperfect bite. Luckily, all of us are growing new bodies day by day, so I enjoy my time with **Dr. Daniel Olsen** making sure I'm growing in the right directions with functional connections between all the parts of my skeleton. The hands-on bodywork includes Dr. Dani's fingers in my mouth toward the end of every session. I can honestly say, she practices mouthbodywork!

I always look forward to this part of the session in my mouth because it invariably is followed by an instantaneous clear-headedness. An ability to take a deep breath. And a deep relaxation of all my muscles (including eye muscles) to allow my entire skeleton to realign in a completely supported and calm state. And I mean *calm*. As in very slow brain wave frequency—theta dipping into delta—sort of in and out of waking consciousness during parts of the session.

Neuroscientists describe this state as a *resting state of functional connectivity* in which seemingly disparate parts of the brain pulse electrically when you're completely relaxed doing nothing. It's much easier to come into realignment in this state—in your physical body, but also in your emotional and mental body. Feeling balanced throughout your whole self feels divine.

Mouth Breathing, Snoring and Mouth Taping

A misaligned jaw and bite can cause some people to suffer from mouth breathing instead of proper nasal breathing through the nostrils, which can also lead to snoring at night. Be aware that mouth breathing and snoring are not only a nuisance, they are also less healthy for the person than normal nasal breathing and can affect how much oxygen you are getting into your lungs during waking and during sleeping. If the problem is not from sinusitis or a structural issue with the nasal passages, consult with a structural dentist to get help correcting your bite. The dentist may recommend a night guard to assist you, or mouth taping where you use small pieces of skin-safe tape on your lips to cue your jaws to stay in alignment. Or your dentist may want to do an overall analysis of your bite using 3D imaging to see what is causing the blockage. If mouth breathing and snoring at night are causing you to lose sleep or are causing sleep apnea, you will want to get to the bottom of the issue and find a resolution because lack of sleep is a precursor to many chronic conditions of ill health.

Resources

If you like to see dental images including clinical images,
go to Google images and search for these keywords to
see plenty of examples of topics covered in this chapter.
If seeing clinical images makes you stressed, no worries.
Skip the images and keep reading to learn how to take
action to support better oral-systemic health.

- *Pacifier and palate deformation*

- *Misaligned bite*

- *Scoliosis after orthodontics*

CHAPTER 8

Daily Mouthbody Self-Care

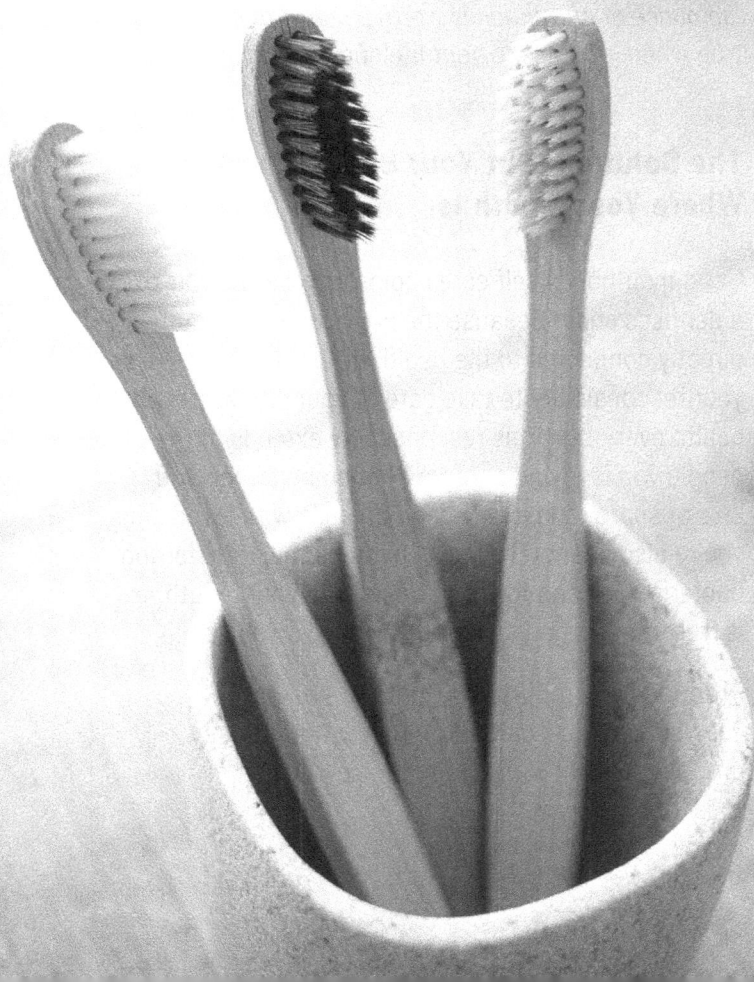

The Problem: Focusing on Treatments Rather Than Prevention

Dental treatments come after there's already a problem in your mouth, but what about preventing those problems from happening in the first place? Of course, when you already have a problem, you want the best oral-systemic dentist you can find. However, the best mouthbody self-care you will ever receive in this lifetime will come from you, in the choices you make every day. The old adage, *"an ounce of prevention is worth a pound of cure"* is really true when it comes to your lifelong mouthbody health.

The Solution: Put Your Body Where Your Mouth Is

Good mouthbody self-care begins long before you sit in a dentist's chair. Because the health of your mouth is directly connected to the health of the rest of you, it's your responsibility to take care of your oral-systemic health every day. This responsibility extends to the people you love and care for. Remember, when you kiss or share food, drinks, and utensils with loved ones, you're also sharing your oral microbiome, transferring bacteria back and forth, so make sure your mouth is free of pathogenic microbes when you share.

Practice daily mouthbody self-care as part of your general self-care plan. Below are 12 daily practices easily within reach for everyone.

12 Mouthbody Healthcare Practices for Lifelong Oral-Systemic Health

1. Kiss Sugar Goodbye

- Eliminate refined sugar from your daily diet and you will reap immediate positive results in your systemic wellbeing. Refined sugar feeds harmful bacteria and fungus in your mouth, contributing to tooth decay and gum disease and contributing to candida overgrowth in your gut. Be rigorous, even a little sugar every day increases your risk of a wide variety of health problems. If you drink alcohol on a daily basis, you'll need to take a sober look at that habit—alcohol is *a lot of sugar.*

- Consider replacing sugar in drinks and baked foods with *xylitol,* a natural sugar substitute that looks like white sugar granules but is made from the bark of birch trees. Xylitol kills caries-causing bacteria and yeast fungus (these microbes eat but cannot digest the bark) but passes through the body without an issue. It's a great way to satisfy a sweet tooth while promoting better mouthbody health. An article published in the *Journal of the American Dental Association* recommends putting a spoonful in your mouth to dissolve and swish for a couple minutes, 2-5 times a day. Swishing longer is less effective than swishing more often. You can also buy xylitol gum, toothpaste, or mouthwash.

- If you need some coaching to help you detach from a sugar, alcohol or comfort food habit, read my book ***FAST THERAPY: A 10-Day Self-Healing Program for Mindbody Change*** to start making healthy changes that matter to your intestines, liver and colon but also to your mouth, gums and teeth. The program will teach you how to do a 10-day nutritional liquid fast designed to flush out toxic waste, restore better gut and oral health, and help you break sugar cravings.

2. Keep Your Mouth Hydrated between Meals

- Dry teeth are more susceptible to cavities, so keep your mouth hydrated with alkaline filtered water or spring water throughout the day. Our teeth naturally demineralize and remineralize before, during and after meals. While chewing, our mouth is naturally more acidic, and this can demineralize tooth enamel. After eating, if your mouth has enough bioavailable water and minerals, your teeth will naturally remineralize before your next meal. Get in sync with this natural process and help yourself out by sipping mineral water, green tea and herbal teas between meals (rather than with meals). Avoid sugary or acidic drinks that can leave you with a dry mouth later, weaken your tooth enamel, and feed pathogenic microbes. Sip water throughout the day to keep your mouth moist; *drink before you're thirsty.*

3. Get Enough Vitamin D3 & K2 to Support Healthy Tooth and Bone Growth

- Healthy teeth and bones (I say "and" but really your teeth are bones) need Vitamin D3 metabolized from sunlight on your skin along with Vitamin K2 to shuttle calcium out of your blood where it gunks up artery walls, and into your teeth and bones. Get outside to exercise in the sun whenever you can. Weight bearing exercise triggers bone growth, and sunlight fuels the energy to metabolize calcium and magnesium into healthy bone and teeth. Remember to eat your dark leafy greens for more Vitamin K.

- For supplementation, my favorite brands to get more Vitamin D especially in winter months include *Designs for Health* D-EVAIL 10K Highly Bioavailable Vitamin D with K1, K2 and GG for optimal calcium absorption, or *Metagenics* Vitamin D3 + K, or *Dr. Mercola's* Vitamins D3 & K2. All softgels.

4. Consume Enough Minerals to Remineralize Your Teeth

- Remember your teeth are constantly repairing and regrowing under the wear and tear of chewing your food whenever you eat. Each tooth demineralizes in the acidic environment of saliva during chewing, and then afterwards remineralizes if enough water and minerals are available. So teeth are continuously demineralizing and remineralizing in a cycle. If you want strong and flexible bones and teeth, you also need a 2:1 ratio of calcium and magnesium—often called the *"forgotten nutrient for dental health"* because the two minerals need to be available to teeth and bones *together,* and magnesium is the most common nutrient deficiency in the U.S.

- A diet rich in organic whole foods grown in mineral-rich farm soils provides the necessary nutrients to keep your teeth and bones strong. Choose foods high in calcium and magnesium such as nuts, seeds, dark leafy greens, and fatty fish. Your best source of Vitamin D is sunshine on your skin. You can source additional Vitamin D in raw butter and dairy, but it has to be raw—once pasteurized (heated) the natural Vitamin D is no longer bioavailable (hence why commercial pasteurized milk often is marketed as "fortified" with synthetic Vitamin D, as if that were a plus). Avoid processed foods that can deplete your body of the minerals it needs every day, such as refined sugar, flour and corn syrup, and reduce your consumption of red meat—which takes a really long time to digest and for the waste to be eliminated.

- For supplementation, stick with brands you trust. In my experience, cheaper is not better when it comes to buying nutritional supplements. My favorite brands for mineral supplementation include *Beam Minerals'* liquid Micro-Boost Complete Mineral Supplement, *Maximum Living* MineralRich plus Aloe, *Solgar's* liquid Calcium Magnesium Citrate with Vitamin D3 and natural blueberry flavor, and *Trace Minerals* Trace Mineral Drops.

5. Avoid Fluoride in Tap Water and Toothpaste

- Industrial grade fluoride is a waste product of the fertilizer industry and is sold to municipal water treatment facilities under the pretense that it is good for our teeth. Fluoride is absorbed like calcium into teeth and bones, but unlike calcium that makes bones and teeth strong and flexible, fluoride makes bones and teeth strong and brittle, leading to more fractures over time. High levels of fluoride are also known to cause neurotoxicity in adults associated with negative impacts on memory and learning, and those impacts are even more serious for vulnerable developing children and teens. Fluoride is also absorbed like calcium into the pineal gland in the brain, causing calcification of the gland, and disrupting healthy melatonin regulation.

- An easy remedy if your local tap water is treated with fluoride is to use filtered water or spring water for brushing your teeth, rinsing your mouth, and drinking, and use a shower filter or bath ball filter for bathing. Obviously, you'll need to choose a natural toothpaste that is fluoride free.

6. Scrape Your Tongue Every Morning

- Start each day by scraping your tongue with a metal scraper or spoon to remove the mucus film of waste, bacteria and yeast that can accumulate and get pushed to the surface overnight. Why swallow all that gunk down and then have to detox it again tomorrow? Help your mouthbody eliminate this waste more easily and quickly. Follow tongue scraping with xylitol swishing for added cleansing. Choose a metal tongue scraper over cheaper plastic ones to reduce exposure to microplastics—if they're in your mouth you're going to swallow them down into your gut and from there they can get everywhere.

7. Carry Floss

- Flossing is just as important as brushing, if not more so, because it helps manage plaque buildup between teeth and at the gum line. Carry floss with you. To protect vulnerable tooth enamel right after a meal when your mouth is acidic and your teeth are naturally demineralized, it's better to floss between teeth than brush. Instead, brush your teeth later when your teeth have remineralized. My favorite floss by far is **Clean Planeterra's Natural Silk Dental Floss** packaged in a glass container. This Green America certified, zero landfill solution, renewable materials packaged floss made from just pure silk thread and candelilla wax eliminates plastic floss and packaging from both your mouth and the environment.

8. Choose Natural Toothpastes and Toothbrushes

- Choose a natural toothpaste made with neem, bentonite clay, baking soda or charcoal without harmful additives like fluoride, sodium lauryl sulfate (a sudser), and synthetic antibacterial agents.

- The story of triclosan provides a cautionary tale regarding additives. Triclosan was on the market for several decades first appearing in the early 1960s as a pesticide. It then became widely used in consumer products like soaps, toothpastes, antiseptic washes, deodorants, shower gels and dishwashing liquids as an antibacterial compound until it was banned (along with 18 other antimicrobial agents) by the FDA in 2016 from soaps—though it remained in Colgate Total toothpaste until 2019. Think how many tens of millions of Americans exposed themselves to this toxic chemical compound every day for all those decades before triclosan was banned. Its harmful effects include increased risk of global bacterial resistance to antibiotics, hormone disruption (it was found in breastmilk, urine and blood plasma) as well as its accumulative ecotoxic effects in the environment. Be careful what you put in your mouthbody! Decide for yourself how much you can trust the FDA.

- Choose bamboo toothbrushes with natural bristles to reduce plastic landfill waste and to keep microplastics out of your mouth.

- Sanitize your toothbrush after each use (there are many good toothbrush sanitizers on the market including compact travel models) and replace your toothbrush with a new fresh one every 3 months.

9.   Avoid Overusing Antibiotics

*   Antibiotics kill both pathogenic and beneficial bacteria in your mouth and gut, leading to imbalances that contribute to chronic mouthbody ill health. Use antibiotics *only when absolutely necessary,* and then follow up with prebiotics and probiotics to help restore a healthy microbiome. If you've already experienced rounds and rounds of antibiotics in your life, you might want to consider using **beta glucans** to help your immune system out while stepping away from the antibiotics.

10. Oil Pulling

*   Swish a spoonful or two of coconut oil or sesame oil in your mouth for 10-20 minutes. Oil pulling helps detoxify the mouth, soothe the gums, and mineralize the teeth. After oil pulling, spit the oil into the trash, not the sink. It will stop it up.

11. Remove Toxic Substances and Chronic Infections from Your Mouthbody

*   Toxic substances in your mouth like mercury fillings and other mixed metals in dental work can expose your whole body to daily stress and inflammation. Work with a skilled systemic dentist to identify and remove these toxic substances from your mouthbody to reduce the risk of long-term effects on your systemic health.

12. Invite Your Dentist and Doctor to Talk to Each Other

- Dental and medical health are interconnected, so encourage your doctor and dentist to collaborate on your care. By sharing information, they can better address both dental and systemic health issues at the same time. Make sure you make that conversation easy by providing emails and phone numbers and inviting your practitioners to team up on your behalf. Schedule a conference call to get the ball rolling.

Resources

If you like to see dental images including clinical images, go to Google images and search for these keywords to see plenty of examples of topics covered in this chapter. If seeing clinical images makes you stressed, no worries. Skip the images and keep reading to learn how to take action to support better oral-systemic health.

- *How to tongue scrape*

- *How to floss*

- *How to brush teeth*

CHAPTER 9

Finding an Oral-Systemic Dentist

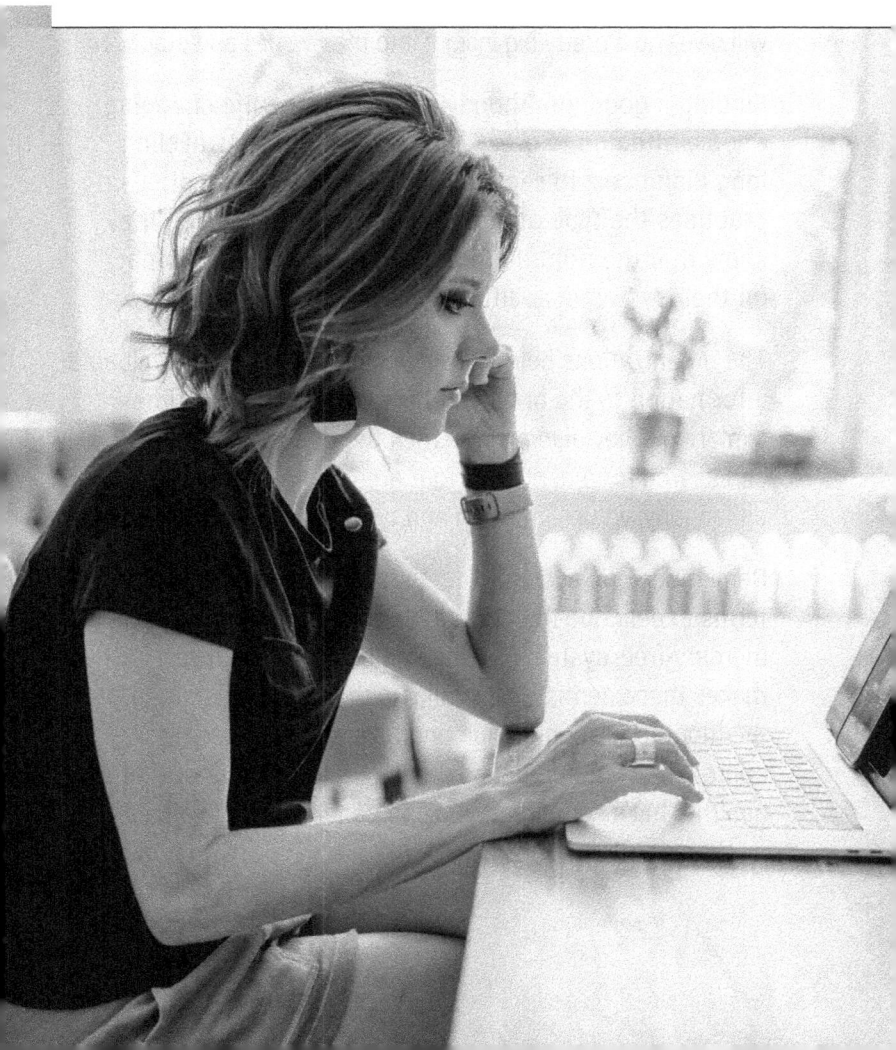

Online Resources

There are many, many professional dental organizations that promote safer, less invasive, more holistic approaches to dentistry with a focus on overall systemic health. It is important that you know about these organizations because they promote dental practices that are better for your overall health. When searching for a systemic dentist for yourself and your family, ask about the professional organizations the dentist belongs to. That will give you a pretty big insight into their values and practices.

Finding a good mouthbody dentist can be life changing. People often go to great lengths, sometimes traveling long distances, to see a biological or holistic dentist who practices the type of dentistry they need, because they know that the right dentist can have a profound impact on their systemic health for many years to come.

The organizations below have websites that provide valuable information to the public and are well worth your time exploring. They also provide member directories where you can search for a dentist in your area and read about the philosophy, values, mission and type of services they practice.

Remember, oral-systemic dentists might use different terms to describe their practice—such as holistic, biological, mercury-free, systemic or minimally-invasive. However, what makes these dentists all similar is that they understand the mouthbody connection and take an oral-systemic approach to your dental health in relation to your overall health. That's something you can genuinely smile about.

Dental Organizations That Value a Systemic Approach to Mouthbody Healthcare

If you are looking for a dentist, I recommend you dedicate some time researching these organizations and searching the dentists listed in their directories *before* you face a dental emergency. It's always better to find a systemic dentist who aligns with your mindbody health goals *before* there's a problem. Find a dentist you feel good about teaming up with and schedule a consultation.

- American Academy of Ozonotherapy **(AAO)**

- Holistic Dental Association **(HDA)**

- International Academy of Biological Dentistry and Medicine **(IABDM)**

- International Academy of Oral Medicine and Toxicology **(IAOMT)**

- Mercury-Safe Dentists **(MSD)**

- World Alliance for Mercury-Free Dentistry **(MFN)**

- American Academy for Oral Systemic Health **(AAOSH)**

Questions to Ask When Searching for a Systemic Dentist

Have these questions handy when you interview a prospective dentist to team up with you to establish and sustain better mouthbody health. You'll know from the answers if you found the right systemic dentist for you.

1. **Trainings?** Does the dentist have specific trainings in areas of your concern? What courses, workshops, or certifications have they completed?

2. **Mercury-Free?** Does the dentist practice mercury-free dentistry?

3. **Mercury Removal Safety Protocol?** Does the dentist know how to remove mercury amalgam fillings safely? What is the safety protocol? Is a dental dam and nasal oxygen mask used? Is the room ventilated? Do the patient, the dentist and the staff wear protective gear?

4. **Holistic Approach?** Does the dentist take an oral-systemic approach to mouthbody health and use minimally-invasive treatments?

5. **Ozone and Other Oxygen Therapies?** Does the dentist use ozone gas, ozonated water, or ozone trays? Are other oxygen therapies available, such as hydrogen peroxide therapy ($H2O2$)?

6. **No-Drill Cavity Options?** Does the dentist offer non-drilling options for treating cavities, such as air abrasion or ozone therapy?

7. **Laser Light therapy?** Does the dentist use red laser light therapy during teeth cleaning to treat periodontal plaque along the gumline?

8. **Biomimetic Materials?** Are biomimetic materials like zirconia used for fillings, caps and posts? Is bio-compatibility testing done?

9. **Root Canals?** Does the dentist discourage root canals due to risk of chronic infection? How does the dentist treat an infected root canal? What treatments does the dentist offer instead of root canals?

10. **Wisdom Tooth Extractions?** Does the dentist avoid unnecessary early wisdom tooth extractions? Are less invasive alternatives considered first?

11. **Cavitations?** Does the dentist know how to treat cavitations or deep focal infections in tooth sockets after tooth extractions?

12. **IV Treatments?** Does the dentist offer IV mineral and vitamin delivery during dental procedures?

13. **References?** Can the dentist refer you to patients who have had similar treatments so you can ask them about their experience?

Give yourself time to find a good systemic dentist to go on your healing journey with. By interviewing dentists and asking these questions *before* you sit in their dental chair, you'll get a clear picture early on about whether a particular dentist is right for you. Take your time choosing your dentist so you can go forward feeling confident that you are mindfully making an informed choice to support your lifelong oral-systemic health.

Be sure to share this book with people in your life who need to know about the mouthbody connection. Sharing is caring. If you found this book helpful, leave a review on Amazon to help the algorithm share out. It matters!

Healing Dental Trauma

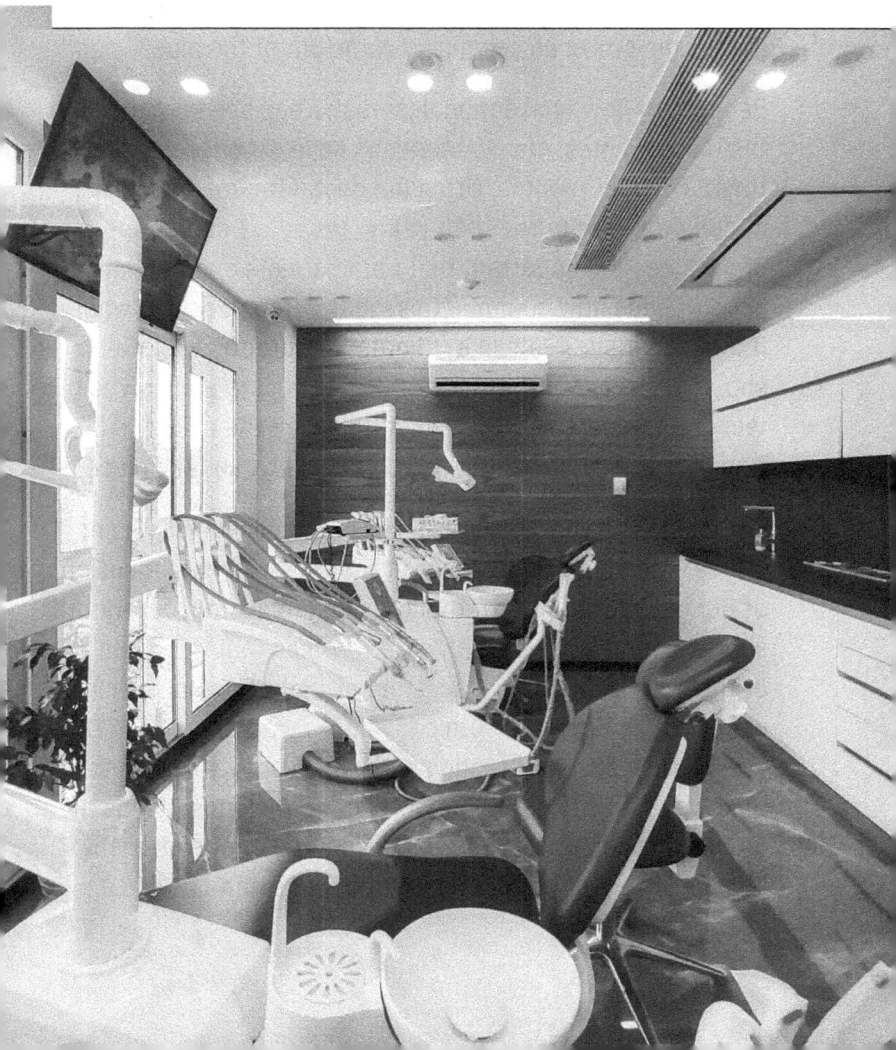

Post traumatic stress (PTSD) is now generally recognized in psychology and psychotherapy and many people are aware that trauma can leave long-lasting effects on our physical, mental and emotional body. The imprint of a traumatic event on the psychology of a person can last long after the original trauma has taken place, creating 'triggers' that can last for years and decades afterward. Once triggered, the release of an intense charge of emotional energy from a body memory stored in a particular part of the body can seemingly come out of the blue.

Because of how conventional dentistry has been practiced in the United States, many Americans have experienced dental trauma in their mouths. Often the dental trauma happens in childhood, or in the teen years, though it can happen at any age. It is important that both patients and dentists acknowledge how common this kind of trauma is and what it looks like and feels like. Clients and practitioners alike should be aware of the signs of dental trauma and how to recognize, treat and prevent it. In this way, the risk of re-traumatization can be reduced and healing can take place.

Our mouth is a very vulnerable part of our bodymind. As an orifice at the boundary between the visceral inside dimension of our being and the external outside dimension, our mouth shares characteristics with other orifices that are some of the most vulnerable places in our body. For this reason, dental trauma in our mouth can cause symptoms of PTSD that deserve special attention and care in order to heal and to prevent. A good oral-systemic dentist who understands the mouthbody connection and who recognizes the relationship between one's physical bodily experience and one's emotional and mental experience is going to be prepared to ease the stress on patients when they sit in the dental chair for a treatment. If you're aware that you have had dental trauma, share your history with your current dentist so you can team up to work together through any triggers or somatic-emotional releases that might come up for you. A good dentist who understand the mouthbody connection will be willing to help you through your healing process.

The best option you have if you have experienced dental trauma from conventional dentistry is to ask for help to remedy the situation if there is still a problem in your mouth from that experience in the past. Whether it is mercury amalgam dental fillings that were placed in your teeth or a root canal treatment on a dead tooth or an empty tooth socket from a wisdom tooth extraction that has become infected and continues to negatively affect your systemic health in the present, or misaligned fillings or crowns that changed the structure of your bite and left you in chronic neck and shoulder pain—whatever happened to you in the past, you have a choice in the present. Rather than continue to live with that dental trauma, find a good oral-systemic dentist who can help you bring peace to your mouthbody by taking care of the root of the problem.

Many people who have been traumatized by a dentist will avoid going to the dentist in the future, but that often means they cannot fix the traumatic wound in their mouth that may be ongoing and causing so much pain and suffering and possibly jeopardizing their long-term health outcomes. To heal a traumatic wound or injury in your mouth, ask for help. Just make sure you ask a dentist who actually knows how to help you. If you search for an oral-systemic dentist, you will find one, because they're out there. You just need to be clear about what you need and what you're looking for as an informed, conscious consumer, and be willing to speak up. Start by scheduling a simple consultation, and ask a friend or relative to go with you.

Be prepared that when you choose oral-systemic dentistry over conventional dentistry, there may be costs involved that your dental insurance won't pay for (if you have dental insurance). That's actually a good sign that you're on the right track! Because the up-front costs for quality dental materials and technologies mean you're not on the *drill it, fill it, bill it'* roller coaster that will have you back in the dentist's chair year after year and decade after decade spending more and more money until you end up one day in dentures. Cost-effective doesn't mean cheap. Ask the oral-systemic dentist that you find about a payment plan if you need one, because they all have them, and put your money where your mouth is. Trust that your lifelong mouthbody healthcare is worth every penny of your investment.

Other books by Camilla Griggers:

BECOMING-WOMAN

FAST THERAPY

ABOUT THE AUTHOR

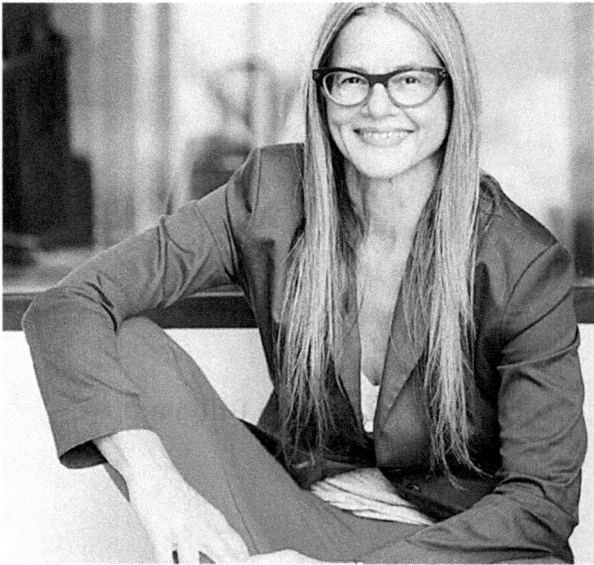

Photo by Anja Epkes at anjaepkes.com

Camilla Griggers, PhD is a feminist cultural theorist, somatic therapist and educator, and holistic health consultant. Her books and articles integrate cultural analysis and psycholinguistics with somatic therapies for an innovative perspective on preventive self-care and healthcare. A university professor for twenty years before pivoting into the holistic healing arts, she applies her broad knowledge base to educating the public about preventive self-care practices easily within reach that reduce the risk of chronic mindbody illness and support the development of lifelong wellbeing. She lives in Santa Monica, California by the beach where she enjoys writing educational and inspirational books about holistic health that cross the mindbody and mouthbody divide.

* 9 7 8 1 9 6 2 9 8 4 9 4 2 *